Thomas Hoby Earl
of Stair *

Jno. Stair

ALLERGIES:
Questions and Answers

Doris J Rapp MD
and
A W Frankland MD

HEINEMANN HEALTH BOOKS
London

First published 1976
© Doris Rapp and A W Frankland 1976
ISBN 0 433 10881 9

"Heinemann Health Books" are published
by William Heinemann Medical Books Ltd.

Photoset by Seventy Set, Ltd, London, and
printed by Redwood Burn Ltd., Trowbridge and Esher

Contents

Preface

This book is written with the idea that most patients have many unanswered questions in relation to their specific allergies. Allergic complaints are often little understood by patients because explanations are so time-consuming and repetitious. Therefore, we have set out to answer many of the questions that patients have asked about allergies.

To have an allergy surely is not pleasant but, fortunately, there are a few good things about this type of medical problem. For example, the onset of allergies can sometimes be prevented or delayed, if the patient knows what to avoid. The treatment of allergies is often essentially the *same,* regardless of which part of the body is affected; i.e., nose, lungs, eyes, skin, etc. The *same* methods of treatment often help infants, children or adults. Success or failure depends to a great degree, not so much upon the physician, but upon the determination of the patient to follow his doctor's recommendations. Allergy treatment does not always require allergy injections.

We explain how each type of allergy may be investigated and treated. There are over 500 questions and it is our earnest hope that not only have we asked questions that you would ask, but that we have answered them in a helpful way. The book is written to have an international appeal, but different countries, races and religions have different ways of living. Not only is the allergic environment different, but home construction, heating and foods and even the spelling of words are different. Yet, basically, in allergy everything is amazingly similar.

An allergy can be compared to having a nail in your shoe causing a sore on your foot. The treatment is not an ointment for the sore, but removal of the nail. Some of the allergy "nails" are amazingly simple to remove. We suggest you read the first chapter as an introduction and, thereafter, find the question and answer that concerns your problem. You may find that some symptoms you suspected, as well as some you didn't suspect, might be due to allergy.

We hope that you will know more about your allergies after reading this book. Much can be done to help a complaint that is allergic so we hope this book will help you to understand more about how to recognise and treat your allergic problem and why your physician arrives at a decision about its management.

As with most medical advice, it is best to check with your physician for he alone knows your personal health problems. He can guide you and adapt your allergy care to your specific needs so that the best therapy for your allergy problems can be found.

CHAPTER ONE

Introduction

Which parts of a person's body can be affected by allergies?
Almost any part of the body. The portion of the body which is affected is called a shock organ. Common ones are the nose and eyes (hay fever), the skin (eczema and nettle rash (welts), chest (asthma or wheezing), intestines, or ears.

A single substance can cause allergies in multiple areas or different allergenic substances could cause symptoms in several shock organs. For example, dust can cause hay fever and asthma in one person, while in another individual, dust may cause hay fever, while grass pollen may cause asthma.

1. Chest allergies are sometimes manifested by recurrent coughing which does not respond to the "usual" cough remedies. Asthma is only one cause of wheezing. Usually wheezing means that the individual has more difficulty breathing out than he does breathing in. As he expires or blows the air from his lungs, there is a whistling sound within his chest. If asthma is severe, there may be wheezing during both breathing in and breathing out. (See Chapter 3).

2. Nose allergies are characterized by thin watery mucus, stuffiness, snorting sounds, sniffling, sneezing-in-series, throat-clearing, or an itchy nose. (See Chapter 2).

3. Skin allergies are usually manifested in three major forms:
    a. The first is eczema or atopic dermatitis which is a rash in the creases of the arms or legs or on the back of the neck. (See Chapter 4).
    b. Nettle rash or welts – these are manifested in itchy swellings near the surface of the skin and look like mosquito bites. There is another type which can cause more extensive swelling which is not associated with itching. This can affect larger areas of the body such as the lips, eyes, entire face or arms and is called angioedema. (See Chapter 5).
    c. Contact dermatitis – these are tiny itchy little blisters which are located on the skin in the area which came in contact with the offending substance. It is very common on the hands.

4. Eye allergies usually affect both eyes at the same time and typically cause itching, watery secretions, and redness to occur on the white portion of the eyes (conjunctiva). (See Chapter 2).

5. Intestinal allergies are often the cause of abdominal pain or discomfort, nausea or an upset stomach, problems with bowel movements, or an excessive amount of mucous or intestinal air either in the form of belching or rectal gas.

6. Ear allergies can be noted in the form of an intermittent or constant hearing loss due to the abnormal accumulation of fluid behind an eardrum. Ear allergies can cause dizziness if the inner ear is affected. The outer ear canal is sometimes affected by contact with allergenic substances and this can cause a rash or discharge near the ear opening. (See Chapter 6).

7. Rare forms of allergy might affect the central nervous system causing recurrent headaches, fatigue, hyperactivity, convulsions, changes in disposition such as depression or feelings of anxiety or agitation. Sometimes allergies affect the blood or blood vessels causing various types of bleeding within the skin or the body. Allergies rarely affect the urinary system causing kidney or bladder problems. Sometimes vaginal irritation or itching, a patchy or a spotty tongue (geographic tongue), swelling of the joints, and recurrent cold sores or sores on the lips can be due to allergy. (See Chapter 12).

What are the common causes of allergies?

Allergies can be caused by innumerable substances. Many persons are allergic to things inside their home or to foods which are eaten. These often cause allergies at any time of the year. Others are allergic to things in the outside air and may have problems only during certain seasons of the year. Unfortunately approximately half of all adults who have asthma, wheeze for unknown reasons.

What causes year-round allergies?

This type of allergy often occurs every day or "on and off" throughout the year. The major causes are house dust (mainly due to mites), stuffing of furniture (kapok linters, cotton linters, or hair), mould spores or algae, wool, fur or feathers, pets (hair, dandruff and saliva), debris from insects (mites, cockroaches, beetles, etc.) and perfumed or nice-smelling substances (bubble bath, body oil or powder, scented toilet or facial tissues, body deodorant aerosols, perfumes, or lotions). (See Chapter 2).

How can you detect an allergy due to something in your home?

Home allergies are probable if you are slightly worse during the colder months of the year when indoors and somewhat better in the warmer months when outdoors. This is also true if you are better when you are on vacation, visiting friends, at work, or away from home. Symptoms may be worse when cleaning, remodelling, moving to another home or doing anything within the home which exposes you to excessive dust.

Although someone may be better when he is away from home indicating something at home is at fault, the fact that he is *not* better when away does not mean his home is not related to his allergies. If your problem is due to a pet or feather pillow which you take wherever you go, your allergy problems go with you. If the place you visit is as dusty as your home, the same may be true.

How can you tell if you have a food allergy?

If a patient's symptoms seem to be the same regardless of where the patient happens to be or what he is doing, it is possible that the problem is related to a food. If the problem dates back to early infancy, it is often related to a food which is eaten early in infancy such as milk, wheat, or possibly eggs. If the problem occurs every day, it would tend to indicate that a food eaten every day may be at fault rather than one which is seldom eaten.

If your allergic symptoms are *not* present when you are not eating because of a digestive upset, this could point to a food allergy. Allergic symptoms which disappear when someone is fasting, for example during a religious observance, suggests a food allergy. (See Chapter 19).

What causes seasonal allergies?

The causes would vary depending upon the location in which a person lives. The first substance to cause difficulty after the cold season would be the various tree pollens, the next would be grass pollens and this is closely followed by mould spores and weed pollens. The exact pollination times for various localities are listed on page 260. Grasses tend to pollinate in the late afternoon, while weeds pollinate in the early morning hours (about 4 a.m.).

In relation to trees, each type pollinates and causes symptoms for a short period of one to three weeks each year. The time when a specific tree will pollinate in any particular area is rather consistent and each year pollen will be noted within a few days of the time when it pollinated in previous years. Sometimes trees of the same type will repeatedly pollinate at slightly different times although they are located relatively close to one another. Leaves which fall from trees can become mouldy and cause allergies at that time.

What is pollen?

Pollen is a plant airborne sperm-like substance. Inconspicuous green and drab plants produce plentiful amounts of airborne pollen causing allergies. A single plant can produce many tablespoons of pollen which has the appearance of a fine yellowish powder. Individual pollen granules vary from about 10 to 30 microns in size. A micron is one-thousandth part of a millimeter. There are approximately 25 millimeters to an inch. Different types of pollen can be examined under the microscope and identified.

Can pretty coloured flowers be the cause of allergies?

Most pretty coloured flowers do not cause allergies because they attract insects. Brightly coloured flowers have heavy sticky pollen which is spread by bees as they flit from plant to plant. If flowers are brought very close to the nose or are shaken when arranged, it is possible to breathe the pollen and to have allergic symptoms.

Patients who have weed allergies sometimes, however, have an unusual sensitivity to certain flowers such as daisies, chrysanthemums, zinnias or marigolds.

Persons who handle dried flowers can have symptoms because of moulds which are on them. Spraying flowers with paints or chemicals can cause difficulty. Cocoons and bark can also cause symptoms.

Is it possible to move away from pollens or mould spores?

This would be extremely difficult because most countries have some form of green foliage which pollinates. It is possible to move away from a specific type of pollen which is located in certain areas of a country but the move would probably expose that person to other allergenic pollens which could cause a new sensitivity to develop.

Sometimes people who have allergies are very upset because there are fields of weeds and plants near their home. Pollen and mould spores are very light and can blow for miles on windy days. It is unrealistic to attempt to eliminate nearby fields in an effort to diminish pollen contact. If, however, someone is allergic to the type of tree pollen found immediately outside his home, he might consider planting a type of tree which did not cause allergies. In general, if someone lives in rural country areas, there are more problems with pollens. If one lives in urban areas. Pollens are still evident and pollution could be a significant problem.

Do some substances cause allergies at one time and not at another?

Yes, for example a person can be allergic to grass pollen but not have difficulty when there is relatively little grass pollen in the air. At a certain point, however, there could be enough grass pollen in the air so that symptoms occur. Each person who has allergies to grass pollen has a threshold or tolerance for that particular pollen. You can be exposed to a substance to which you are allergic and not have symptoms merely because you have not been exposed to enough of it.

Most people are allergic to more than one substance. Whether a person has symptoms or not at any particular time would depend upon the number of these substances which were in the person's contact or surrounding at a particular time. An extremely large exposure to only one of

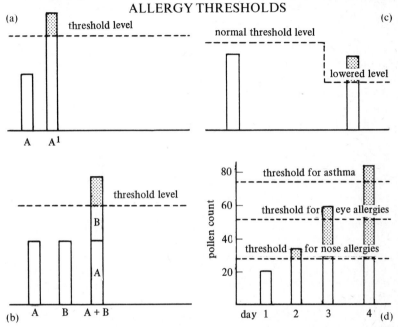

ALLERGY THRESHOLDS

(a) illustrates why the same substance causes allergies on some but not all occasions. A = a little dust, or cat, or pollen. A^1 = an excessive amount of dust, cat or pollen. A causes no symptoms because the total exposure is below the threshold level. A^1 causes symptoms because the amount is greater than the patient can tolerate. This situation could arise from cleaning a dusty basement or when a cat is shedding.

(b) illustrates why a little of two allergenic substances, A or B, causes no allergy but if a patient is exposed to both A and B at the same time, they add to more than the patient's threshold tolerance, and symptoms occur. A plus B is too much, while either alone is not excessive.

(c) illustrates why a patient can ordinarily tolerate a certain exposure of something such as dust without having allergic symptoms. Infection, exercise or fatigue, emotional upsets, chilling, or exposure to irritants such as smoke can lower a normally high threshold so that the usual exposure to an allergenic substance becomes excessive and symptoms are produced.

(d) On day 1, there are no symptoms because the pollen count is below the patient's threshold levels. On day 2, the patient has nose symptoms of allergy because the pollen count is above this threshold level. On day 3, the patient has nose and eye allergic symptoms because the pollen count is now above both these threshold levels. On day 4, this same patient has nose, eye, and chest symptoms of allergy because the pollen level has exceeded these threshold tolerances for this patient.

them could cause symptoms, or small exposure to many allergic substances all at once could cause similar difficulty. A common example is a problem created by pets. If a dog has recently been bathed and is not shedding, the pet might not cause symptoms, but if the same dog has much dandruff and is losing its hair, it could cause symptoms especially if the dog were cuddled or hugged.

Is it possible for a person to detect the cause of his allergies without a physician's help?

Although it is surely not always possible to determine the cause of an allergic problem, sometimes it is. If a person is well and *suddenly* develops hay fever, asthma, an allergic cough, hives, or eczema, he must think about what preceded the allergic symptoms. Repeatedly ask yourself: Why today and not yesterday? Why this afternoon and not this morning? At the *very first evidence* of difficulty, the individual should immediately sit down and write a diary of EVERYTHING placed in his mouth, or any unusual contacts during the previous 12 hours or so. The cause may be obvious, such as an insect sting, contact with a pet, or an infection. At other times, in spite of your efforts, you may not be able to determine what caused a particular episode. Do not be disturbed if this happens. It may not be possible. Some types of allergy are not caused by obvious exposure to something different. If, however, you never think about what might have caused symptoms, you will surely be less apt to determine offending substances than if you spend time to consider possible factors.

If you keep detailed records and compare the collected information, you may eventually note that red-dyed foods, sitting in a certain chair, using some special cosmetics, a visit to a friend's home, or a certain odour within your house always precedes the onset of allergies. If you spend the time to think seriously about the cause, it is possible that you may greatly help yourself and your physician. Once you know what is causing your allergies, you know what needs to be avoided. Your physician may be able to provide added insight into hidden or concealed forms of some allergenic contacts.

Emotions, infections, fatigue and exercise can all trigger allergic symptoms, but the causative factors are often something unusual that has been breathed or something which has been touched or eaten.

One must, however, be wary because the cause is not always obvious. It is possible to have symptoms on several occasions which seem to be unrelated but actually are. For example, a cherry-flavoured beverage, a cherry-flavoured candy, a cherry-flavoured gelatin and a cherry-flavoured medicine could all cause difficulty on different occasions. Unless one were observant and kept detailed records, one might not realize that it was the cherry flavour or the red dye causing symptoms because the actual item was not the same in each instance.

Are allergies increasing?

There seems to be little doubt that more people are now aware of the fact that they have allergies than ever before. There, however, are many individuals who have mild or even moderate forms of allergy and are not aware that this is the cause of their problem.

There is a general opinion among allergists that one reason for the increase in allergies is the fact that everyone is being exposed to more potentially allergenic substances than ever before. For example, food additives have increased at a tremendous rate with the result that persons are now becoming allergic to items which simply weren't part of our diet 30 to 40 years ago. Air pollution is a contributing factor and this has increased markedly during the past few years in many areas of the world.

How can you tell when you should see an allergist?

If you find that your symptoms interfere with normal activities such as sleep, school, work, or play, your allergies should be evaluated by a physician who is specifically trained or interested in allergies. If a person has only one wheezing episode with an infection it does not mean that an allergist is needed. If the wheezing, however, becomes a recurrent problem or if allergic symptoms are severe, an allergist should be seen. It is indeed possible for allergies to make some persons, especially children, prone to recurrent colds or infection.

Having one single allergy does not necessarily mean that more allergies cannot develop. An allergist may help to prevent or delay the occurrence of new allergies under certain circumstances. For example, an infant who has eczema has a 50 per cent chance of developing other forms of allergies in the future. A child who has eye and nose symptoms of allergies during a weed pollen pollinating season has approximately a 40 per cent chance of subsequently developing asthma or wheezing during that weed pollen pollinating season. Measures should, therefore, be taken in some patients to prevent or delay the occurrence of future problems. (See Chapter 17).

Can you tell if you are apt to develop allergies?

There are a number of characteristics which would indicate that a certain person would be more apt to develop multiple allergic problems than someone else. The *fewer* of the following which an individual has, the better:

1. A strong family history of allergies – many relatives who have this type of problem.
2. A typical allergic appearing face. (See page 2).
3. A personal history of some type of allergy such as hay fever,

asthma, and eczema.
4. Strong evidence of allergies in a person's blood or nose mucus.

What exactly does a physician who treats allergy do?
The initial problem facing the doctor is to determine whether a person's symptoms are truly caused by allergies. Many medical problems can mimic allergies. The physician must, also, determine if the symptoms are serious enough to require a complete and through allergic evaluation. At times the problems are relatively minor and medical advice is all that is necessary.

Most patients who see a physician who treats allergy require some form of medication in order to relieve symptoms. All patients should remember that an allergy can be similar to having a nail in your shoe. The real treatment may not be to apply ointment to the sore on your foot but to remove the nail. The function of the allergist is to find out exactly what is causing the allergic symptoms if possible and to help the patient eliminate these factors. At times, the cause is obvious and avoidance of the offending substance is adequate to eliminate the problem. In many patients some combination of changing the home, diet or environment would be indicated. The allergist can determine whether the cause of the patient's difficulty is most apt to be foods or something in their home. If the home is the major suspect (See page 11), an attempt should be made to make the area in which the person lives much more free of allergenic substances than it has been in the past. At times this method of therapy is entirely successful and within a couple of weeks the patient's symptoms subside completely. In other patients there is incomplete or no improvement indicating that other forms of treatment would be necessary.

The physician may believe that the most likely cause of the patient's problem is a food (See page 12) and dietary trials might be attempted to determine exactly which food or foods were causing difficulties. The degree of success of this form of treatment would vary from patient to patient. It is possible that elimination of the offending food substances could cause complete or partial disappearance of all symptoms, sometimes in a few days or weeks.

If a patient continues to have symptoms in spite of changes in his home and diet, various types of allergy skin or breathing tests would have to be carried out to determine what is causing a particular patient's problems. From allergy skin tests it is possible to prepare a vaccine or extract which can be injected into the patient. The vaccine causes protection to form within the body so that future exposure to offending substances should cause fewer or no symptoms. (See Chapter 10).

Can a person's allergies disappear entirely by changing his home?
This is often the simplest, least expensive, and most rewarding method

of handling an allergic problem. A stuffed toy, dusty furnace, old mattress, feather pillow, or family cat may be the major or sole cause of a particular patient's problems. Improvement following the removal of the offending item can be dramatic. An allergist may be able to determine the major probable cause of someone's allergies at the time of the initial visit. This form of therapy, however, probably would not be adequate if a person had seasonal pollen or mould spore symptoms.

Can a person's allergies disappear by merely changing his diet?

This is very possible especially if the symptoms were first noted in early infancy. Diet might also be the answer for a patient whose family tends to have food allergies. It is not unusual for adults and children to have nose, chest or indigestion-type problems which stop completely once the offending foods are eliminated. The foods which are most apt to cause allergies and how to eliminate them is discussed in Chapter 12.

Is it possible for allergies to disappear if the only treatment is allergy shots?

Some patients do improve if they receive injection treatments with allergy extracts without any consideration of home factors or food. This is particularly true for seasonal pollen allergies.

In some homes it is not possible to eliminate dust, for example, to such a degree that the patient no longer has symptoms. Such a patient might derive more relief of his symptoms if he were given injections of a dust extract in addition to decreasing dust exposure within the home.

It seems foolish to subject someone to testing and injection therapy for many years if the offending substance can easily be eliminated. It is more logical to remove a feather pillow than it is to skin test for feathers and treat someone for this item for many years.

Do all persons who have allergies need extract injection therapy?

No. If the symptoms are mild and infrequent, a person may need only the correct drug to use whenever indicated. If, however, the symptoms are severe and if home changes for allergies and dietary studies aren't indicated or do not help, allergy injection therapy might be indicated. In general, although many patients respond to the type of treatment which has been outlined, it certainly cannot be stated that all patients do. Patients may be helped completely, to a degree, or not at all, regardless of what the allergist does. Fortunately, the latter are a minority.

Why aren't all patients helped by home changes, diets, and allergy injection treatments?

Allergies can be caused by some substances which we do not even know about at the present time. Some allergies are partially or entirely unrelated to exposure and seem to be due possibly to a lack of certain chemicals within the body. When this deficiency is replaced in the form of certain drugs, the patient improves. It is somewhat similar to a diabetic who needs insulin. At this time, we do not understand fully why these chemicals may not be sufficiently abundant in certain allergic individuals. We do not know if this type of problem is inherited or if it can be acquired during one's life. With time and research, we should be able to find more answers concerning why one person is more prone to have allergies than someone else.

If an allergist is not readily available, can you determine what is causing your allergies?

If your symptoms occur each year at the same time when pollens or mould spores are in the air (See page 24), it would probably indicate that you would have to be skin tested and receive treatment for the seasonal substances to which you are sensitive. Your physician could advise you concerning where skin testing could be done. (See Chapter 10) for more details.

If, however, your symptoms occur either intermittently or daily throughout the year and there is no particular pollen season when you seem worse, it is possible that you might be able to detect some of the causes of your allergic symptoms and eliminate them providing your physician *has definitely diagnosed your problem as an allergy.* Chapter 11 details exactly how to eliminate highly allergenic things from your home and Chapter 12 explains how to check for food allergy.

Upon what does improvement of an allergy depend?

The degree of improvement noted in most patients will vary depending upon the age when the allergies began, how severe they are, and how long they have been a problem. In some instances, the allergic person will follow every suggestion and recommendation which is made. These patients are often quickly rewarded by feeling better. Some patients will not carry out relatively simple suggestions. For example, it is very difficult to convince an adult to encase the box springs with plastic, or that a youngster cannot play *directly* on a carpet. Some patients, however, do what is requested but unfortunately their problems persist. Adult asthmatics are sometimes very difficult to treat. In general, their attacks can be controlled but it is not always possible to know what has caused an attack or how to prevent it.

Some individuals continue to have symptoms although everyone knows what is causing the difficulty. A frequent example is the family who has a pet, knows that some member is allergic to it, but refuses to part with it.

There are also some situations which are totally impossible. If a widow has several young children and lives in a very old damp house, it would be difficult for her to make a room allergy-free. Although she had allergies she would probably have to continue to clean her home. To complicate the situation, there might be financial and physical problems which make it impossible for the mother to carry out the doctor's recommendations. This type of situation is most common among the poor and the only solution is to do as much as is sensibly possible.

Another common reason for a poor response to treatment is the fact that it may be very difficult for a family member to avoid certain foods which are commonly eaten. Young children do not understand why certain foods are forbidden and unless there is unity and rapport, the youngster will continually be eating the offending food and be ill constantly because of it. Adults also eat foods to which they are sensitive. They sometimes lack will power, sometimes forget, and sometimes eat offending foods to derive sympathy.

Allergic individuals who are continually exposed to tobacco smoke should expect their problems to persist. Asthmatics who smoke should not expect to feel well or to improve if they will not or can not give up the habit.

Why are allergies difficult to treat?

The basic reason is that an allergy is unlike an infection, such as a sore throat. For the latter, one sees a physician, has an examination, and receives a drug which often eliminates the problem completely within a short period of time. Allergies are more complicated and the treatment is often not solved by taking a drug for a few days. Allergies will often recur repeatedly until the causes of the difficulty are eliminated or the person has received adequate allergy extract therapy.

Many people are helped only after they drastically change their home or what they eat. Allergic persons often need to be skin tested and receive allergy injection treatments for many years. Records must be kept and one must be alert continually to determine the cause of each sudden allergic episode. Methods for treating allergies are sometimes not simple, easy or fast.

Should both parents be present for a child's allergy diagnosis visit?

This would be advisable because parents see their children at different times and notice different things. Every little bit of information will help in the final evaluation and determination of what is causing a child's problems and what is needed to eliminate the problems.

If only one parent can accompany the child, it should be the one who knows most about the youngster.

It is of little value if a friend or a relative is sent with a child. The allergist can always do a thorough physical examination but in the field of allergy, a detailed thorough history is of prime importance and few major decisions can be made without this information.

Can a youngster be too young for allergy treatment?

No. If the symptoms interfere with a youngster's rest or normal activity, the problem should be investigated. Some infants, for example, cannot sleep throughout the night because of a food allergy and once the food is eliminated they rest normally. If a problem is very frequent or severe, regardless of the youngster's age, it is surprising how easy it may be to treat. Very young children or infants can be helped by removing a food, a stuffed animal, a pet, baby oil or powder, or eliminating moulds in a bedroom. Very young children, if they do require skin testing, need only a few tests.

SAMPLE YEAR ALLERGY RECORD

	Jan	Feb	Mar	Apr	May	Jun
Drugs Used to Treat Allergies	N +	W +	W + +	N +	H + +	W + + + N + + S +
Nose, eye, skin	2 ×			1 ×	5 ×	3 ×
Asthma or cough		1 ×	5 ×			19 ×
Infection						1 ×
Known causes					cat	

	Jul	Aug	Sep	Oct	Nov	Dec
Drugs Used to Treat Allergies	N + +	N +	C + +	W + + N + +	Ea +	E + + N + +
Nose, eye, skin	8 ×	1 ×		3 ×	3 ×	9 ×
Asthma or cough			5 ×	7 ×		
Infection			1 ×			
Known causes						egg

Code:
N = nose allergy   + is slight symptoms
W = asthma or wheeze   + + indicates symptoms
H = urticaria or hives   between slight and severe
S = eczema or atopic dermatitis   + + + indicates severe symptoms
Ea = ear allergy   × means times, i.e. medicine
E = eye allergy   used 3 times is 3 ×

An infection indicates a cold or nose, throat, or chest disease caused by germs.

Is there a simplified method of keeping allergy records?
A yearly calendar on one single sheet of paper is shown on page 12. By using a code for the type and severity of symptoms, it is often possible at a glance for an allergist to determine the most likely causes of a patient's symptoms.
Such records require time and thought, but the information might decrease the necessity for injection treatments by months or years. If you know the exact cause of a flare of symptoms, it should be noted on the records.

Does the location of an allergy change as one becomes older?
Allergies do change with age. The portion of the body which is affected can change, as well as the substance which is causing difficulty. Allergic infants initially have eczema (or atopic dermatitis) and colic or belly problems. These problems are mainly caused by foods, but dust moulds, pets or perfumed body powders could be factors. (See Chapter 7).
Eczema or digestion problems are often outgrown by the age of 2 or 3 years. At that time, however, nose symptoms of allergies may occur which can be caused by dust, mould spores, pets, pollens or perfumed substances. A mother may incorrectly interpret this phase as being a "constant slight cold" because the child has minor nose symptoms but is not ill. Later on parents may notice excessive or prolonged coughing with infections. Exertion, exercise or emotional upsets such as laughter, disappointment, or excitement may cause coughing. By the age of 5 years wheezing is frequently noted with infections. Without proper allergy treatment, wheezing can eventually become an intermittent or daily problem which recurs for no apparent reason.
Although the above would be a typical pattern for a very allergic child, many exceptions exist. Some infants have eczema, hay fever and asthma all within the first year of life. Some youngsters stop having eczema when their nose symptoms begin and no longer have nose allergies when the asthma starts. Others can acquire new body locations for their allergies while retaining all of the previous ones. Proper allergy care can not only eliminate a youngster's problem but measures can be taken to help prevent new allergies from developing.

Is it possible to "lose" or "outgrow" allergies?
This can occur but many children are erroneously told that this may happen and their wheezing persists. Studies of children have shown that if hay fever is treated only with antihistamines approximately one third will have symptoms for a few years and then no longer have difficulty. Another third continues to have their hay fever symptoms each year and adjust to the problem. They use antihistamines when needed. The remaining third who develop asthma or allergic coughing most definitely

need an allergist.

Children's allergies frequently change at the time of adolescence, hay fever symptoms in particular can sometimes become worse. (See page 90).

Many persons of all age groups believe that they have "outgrown" their allergies when actually they have only been separated from the cause of their problem. This often happens when a family moves or a youngster leaves home to attend college or marry. The true cause for improvement is often separation from a family pet, dusty home, old mattress, or damp basement.

Some children appear to have lost their allergies. A severe infection, however, in the 30's or 40's triggers an asthmatic episode. Subsequent to this wheezing again may become a constant or frequent problem. Persons who do not develop asthma until they are middle aged or older, may have seasonal problems due to pollens or moulds, or may have daily or intermittent wheezing without obvious cause.

What happens if an asthmatic person does not receive treatment?

The final effect depends upon the severity of the asthma. If the asthma is not severe or frequent, particularly in children, there is a possibility that the wheezing may gradually stop. There are, however, many children and adults who can not tell when they are wheezing. It may be brought to their attention only when they have severe asthma associated with infections.

In general there are many advantages to treating asthma when it first starts, regardless of the patient's age.

1. The earlier asthma is treated, the easier it is to determine the cause and possibly prevent and control future attacks. This diminishes the tendency to chronicity which makes it more difficult to treat.

2. Persons with treated asthma can engage in more normal activity than those who are not. For example, youngsters are able to play, take gym, and compete in sports in a manner similar to other children. Without treatment, however, they become short of breath very quickly and readily realize that they are most unlike other children. It is indeed unfair to deny a youngster the joys of riding a bicycle or playing ball in the hope that this problem will disappear before he is too old to enjoy such activity. Too many children miss a childhood waiting to "outgrow" their allergies.

3. The longer a patient wheezes, the more likely his lungs will eventually become damaged, particularly if he smokes or has frequent infections. It is surprising, however, how often a child's or adult's lung function studies remain entirely normal in spite of many years of asthma.

4. Adults and even children can die from an asthmatic episode. Untreated or improperly treated asthmatics are more apt to develop com-

plications than those who are under the care of a specialist. Without
proper treatment for asthma and at times even with the best and most
modern treatment, disastrous situations can arise.

What should someone know about his allergy problem?
Anyone who has or cares for someone who has allergies must attempt
to learn as much as possible about this medical disease. Asthma and hay
fever can be life-time problems even when cared for by a specialist. A
knowledgeable adult can avoid bringing allergenic substances into the
home and can help the doctor detect possible new causes of allergies.
Alert parents can recognize early allergies in their children and immediately take precautions to help eliminate offending substances and
prevent future problems from arising.

Who should assume the responsibility of caring for an allergic person?
Part of the care must be given by the specialist or the physician in
charge. Allergies, however, are complicated and the parents of allergic
children or persons who have allergies must help to detect and eliminate
allergenic substances. It is essential that both parents, for example, understand as much as possible about their child's allergies because there
are always times when only one parent is home and that parent must be
capable of administering the proper medicines and attempting to ferret
out the cause of that particular episode.
A word of caution should be mentioned concerning parents who leave
their allergic children under the care of someone else while they are on
holiday or away from their home. The person left in charge must *completely* understand exactly when and how to give treatment and when
and who to call if problems arise. Quite often it is assumed that the person in charge is knowledgeable until minor problems become a crisis
because of misunderstanding. Detailed written, as well as verbal,
instructions should be given.

How can anxiety associated with severe asthma be diminished?
It helps if persons near the wheezing individual do not appear
frightened or apprehensive. This is particularly true of parents who
readily convey their feelings to their child. If one parent is more calm
than the other, it is that one who should try to help the frightened ill
youngster. Some people cannot hide their emotions very well and tend to
confirm a child's unwarranted fears. If a parent is concerned or if a person who is wheezing becomes extremely apprehensive, your physician
should be called. In the meantime, appropriate medicines should be
given.

How are families affected if one member has an allergy?
An allergic individual unfortunately can disrupt normal family life.

The type of home, the contents within the home, heating, location of bedrooms, types of cooking, and even outside vegetation might have to be altered because of allergies. Mates or siblings may resent the fact that because someone in the family has allergies they cannot have something they desire, such as a pet.

The tendency to spoil a youngster who has severe allergies is common. The ill child has to be overprotected and at times is poorly disciplined because of his tendency to wheeze, especially when reprimanded. The well children frequently feel "left out" and almost envious of the repeated visits to the doctor and attention which the sick child receives. It is not unusual for brothers and sisters of an asthmatic to become behaviour problems to attract more attention.

Sick youngsters quickly realize their potential power and often exert it in order to satisfy their personal desires. Under these circumstances, it is difficult for parents to set limits, use mature judgement and to say no when it is obviously indicated. Allergic children should be treated as much as possible like other children in the family. If the allergic youngster has been most incorrect, asthma medicine should be given immediately and discipline delayed for approximately 20 minutes. This, however, is not always possible or practical. Under no circumstance should the youngster be allowed to continue unacceptable behaviour merely because he might wheeze.

Adults who have allergies, of course, may have many financial, physical and emotional problems. It helps if a husband or wife understands as much as possible concerning the detection, treatment and prevention of allergies.

Can allergies make you feel guilty?

Adults and children who have asthma often wonder if their problems are imaginary or due to emotions because of statements made by physicians or friends who are unfamiliar with allergy. Similar problems arise if a person has an unusual allergy causing intestinal problems, headaches, or vague nerve complaints. Everyone concerned is greatly relieved when the offending substance, either eaten, inhaled, or touched has been eliminated and the symptoms are gone.

Parents of children, especially if allergies are evident on both sides of the family, feel that the child's problem is their fault. If the allergies are mainly on one side of the family, the blame and subsequent guilt is placed squarely on that parent's shoulders. The other side of the family, however, often has allergies incorrectly diagnosed as sinus infection or a chronic cough. No one is to blame that there are allergies in his family anymore than someone is at fault that his eyes are blue.

Mothers worry if their child does not eat properly, is unhappy or seems unwell, particularly if it is the first born infant. They wonder if they are inadequate; where have they failed? Many become overly compulsive cleaners in their effort to keep their home allergy free. Others become diet experts or food faddists to solve food allergy problems.

Many parents are justifiably concerned about the long term effects of restrictions and limitations recommended to help their child. Most allergists will allow exercise and sports activities if the child is well enough to participate. If he is not, partial restrictions might be suggested such as no outside play if it is rainy or very cold. Only the most severely ill children would be strictly limited. When a patient starts to respond to treatment, more and more activity will be allowed.

Decisions such as whether or not to go to school, visiting friends who have pets, acquiring a pet, or sleeping in the country can cause stress in a parent who wants to make his child happy but keep him well. Check with your physician for help to decide when exceptions should be made and what is reasonable and realistic for you and your family. Your physician will consider all aspects of your child's health and give you his best medical advice.

How long after exposure do allergic symptoms appear?

Certain patients are so sensitive that the mere odour of an item could cause immediate symptoms. (See Chapter 13). If a person, however, were mildly allergic it might require *very close* contact with a particular item for minutes or hours before symptoms occurred. The most difficult allergies to detect are the ones which do not cause immediate symptoms. There may be a gradual build up of the allergenic substance within a person's body. The symptoms appear slowly over a period of several days and gradually become progressively worse making it difficult to detect the time when they started. This is why patients who have allergies should try to develop a detective-type nature.

Is it possible to prevent the development of an allergy?

It certainly is. There are some substances which for unknown reasons frequently cause allergic symptoms. If these are avoided in all forms as much as possible, it is most unlikely that an allergy would develop to these items. Dust which contains house mites cannot be eliminated entirely, but vacuuming stuffed furniture and cleaning mattresses often and well would help to diminish the mite concentration. Parents can decrease the amount of pollen in their home by using air-purifying machines (See page 154). Allergenic furniture stuffing (kapok, feathers, horse hair, wool or cotton stuffing) pets, fur and perfumed substances (See page 139) can be avoided. Foods which frequently cause allergies such as eggs should be avoided during early infancy. Highly allergic youngsters should not eat peanut butter and chocolate every day because these foods so frequently cause difficulty. Although allergic persons are not particularly prone to drug allergy, if several family members have a sensitivity to aspirin or penicillin, these should be avoided by other members. Some forms of air pollution such as cigarette smoke can be avoided or minimized.

How much exposure to a new allergenic substance is needed before symptoms are noted?

The answer depends upon how allergic someone is. Grass pollens in Europe, for example, can cause allergic symptoms within three to five years to some emigrants who have had no grass exposure in the past. In Europe and the British Isles there is essentially no ragweed pollen (See Page 260). If a highly allergic European moved to Canada where ragweed is a major problem, only about two or three years would elapse before ragweed symptoms would be noted. The exposure to ragweed pollen would be limited in most areas of the country to only a few weeks but this substance has a high potential for causing susceptible individuals to develop an allergy to it.

Infants are not unusually allergic to pollens because they have not been exposed for a long enough period of time during the first year of life. A potentially extremely allergic infant could develop pollen allergies by the age of 2 or 3 years.

Some allergists believe that electronic or other air purifiers in bedrooms diminish pollen and dust exposure and possibly delay or prevent the development of allergy.

How can someone be helped if a sudden severe allergic emergency arises?

In general allergic emergencies cause eye, nose, skin and lung or chest symptoms of allergies. Antihistamines would help to control the eye, nose and skin symptoms. Drugs used to treat asthma would control the chest and lung problems.

A common error made when attempting to treat allergic emergencies is to treat only the symptom which occurs initially. If the individual is wheezing, the tendency is to give only an asthma drug. Severe allergic reactions, however, often start in the lungs but within a few minutes the eyes, nose and skin may be involved or the reverse can occur. This can happen even if an individual has never wheezed or had nose and eye allergies before. For this reason, if someone is having an acute severe episode, *both* the antihistamine and drug to treat asthma should be given if these are available. A single correct dose would not be harmful under most circumstances.

An allergic emergency could happen if an exquisitely sensitive person accidentally ate certain foods such as nuts or fish, was stung by an insect or reacted to an allergy extract injection treatment.

What should you do if you can't contact your physician for an emergency?
If an alternate physician is covering for your regular physician, call him. Take care to explain the severity and urgency of the problem. If no physician is immediately available, go to the nearest hospital for emergency treatment.

Can allergies affect work and play?
They surely can. Some women find they cannot clean their homes because of a severe dust or mould allergy. An adult can be allergic to substances which are breathed into his lungs or touched while at work. In general schools are less allergenic than homes but in Chapter 17 a few of the major school allergies are mentioned. Carpeting schoolrooms should be strongly discouraged.

Can allergies affect one's emotions?
Allergies can cause tension, hyperactivity, fatigue, depression and disposition changes. This is most frequently seen in children, but also can occur in adults. Eczema, nose allergies and asthma are typical manifestations of allergy which can interfere with sleep and cause disposition changes. Few realize however that foods or breathed substances may cause excitability or irritability in some people because the brain, for example instead of the nose, is affected by some allergenic substance. If someone is even-tempered and very lovable prior to the onset of allergies and then becomes a most difficult individual, it is possible that allergy treatment will help. A most difficult or emotional child could be that way by nature but it is possible that the youngster, for example, has a milk allergy which dates back to early infancy. (See page 160).
There is a medical condition called the allergic tension-fatigue syndrome. Children with this problem seem very restless, irritable, emotional, tired, tense, sullen and lethargic. They complain of vague body complaints such as aching or not feeling well or frequently cry. Their actions may vacillate between extreme sluggishness and fatigue (despite adequate rest) to irrepressible hyperactivity. Parents may wonder if their child is brain damaged or even if there is a psychiatric problem. The cause of this problem can be a food such as milk, chocolate, eggs or corn or the odour of dust, pollen or perfume. Symptoms may disappear entirely when exposure to the allergenic substances is eliminated.

Does the weather affect allergies?
The weather can alter allergies but the reasons for this are not fully understood. Many asthmatic individuals tend to be worse at night. This could be due to variations in temperature, the position during sleep affecting mucus accumulation in the lungs, or it could be related to normal nightly hormone changes.

Many asthmatics wheeze in the late afternoon or early evening hours. This could be related to sudden drops in temperature. Most asthmatics wheeze when they breathe extremely cold air. Warming the air prior to the time it reaches the lungs by covering the mouth with a scarf or breathing slowly through the nose may decrease this problem. Allergies are often worse when the weather is damp or the barometer falls, especially if the latter happens to be associated with the rapid decline in temperature. Windy days especially during pollen seasons cause increased allergic symptoms. Air pollution, especially thermal inversions, or any condition which keeps air contaminants at ground level, such as a heavy fog, can contribute to allergic symptoms.

Can tobacco smoke cause allergies?

Smoke, tobacco or other types, can be a respiratory irritant in anyone. Persons who have hay fever or asthma are definitely worse when they are exposed to tobacco smoke. Allergic people should not smoke or be near persons who do. Smoking in a closed automobile if a person has allergies would not be advisable.

Can human hair or dandruff cause allergies?

Although this has been suggested, it has never been completely substantiated. Sudden allergic symptoms in beauty parlours or barber shops are frequently due to some substance which has an aroma or is irritating such as hair oils, tonics, sprays, scented powders or dust sweepings. Persons who are exquisitely sensitive to eggs cannot tolerate an egg-containing shampoo.

If a person has allergies whenever he is near someone else it may be caused by scented substances or the type of clothing which is worn. Someone allergic to wool or mohair (goat hair) or to rabbit fur (angora) could have symptoms from contact with someone wearing these items.

Recent studies have shown that a wife can develop such problems as nettle rash (welts), asthma, or hay fever from contact with her husband's semen. Sterility rarely is related to allergy.

Which household chores should allergic persons avoid?

Dust, moulds, furniture stuffing, animals and pollinating vegetation are the major causes of allergies in and about one's home. An allergic person should avoid cleaning places which are musty or dusty. Persons allergic to moulds will have difficulty from gardening. Insecticides, burning leaves or painting could affect some individuals. Those who have eczema should not put their bare hands in strong detergent cleaning solutions. Asthmatics should not shovel snow.

Many persons have allergies at certain times of the year but are better at other times. Try to paint or remodel a home at the good time of the year. It would be very foolish to attempt home improvements at a time when someone were very sick.

Someone who has a grass allergy should not cut the grass although he might be able to cut the grass after he has been adequately treated for this sensitivity. Some patients can tolerate grass cutting when it is not windy or late in the season when the grass is not pollinating heavily.

If an allergic person has to clean a dusty basement or garage, it might be helpful if a mask were worn (See page 261) and he tried to keep his hands as clean as possible and away from his nose.

Persons who have allergies may find that they can't do certain household chores prior to receiving allergy care. These same chores may cause no difficulty once they have been adequately treated.

Any advice for allergic patients when they marry?

Ideally, a person with strong allergies should avoid marrying someone else who has strong allergies. However, this advice is not practical. If two highly allergic persons marry they should attempt to follow the precautions suggested in Chapters 1 and 11 to help prevent their offspring from developing allergies and to decrease their own symptoms. Attempts in this direction, as soon as a couple sets up housekeeping, may be immensely helpful.

How does clinic care compare to private allergy care?

To a great degree the care depends upon the physician who is treating you, regardless of where that physician happens to be located. In some parts of the world hospital clinics may give better treatment than can be obtained in private practice but, in general, this is not true.

Are some people ashamed of having allergies?

Unfortunately many children are upset and attempt to hide the fact they have allergies. Misinformed individuals may believe that all allergies are due to emotional problems and tend to have an unsympathetic attitude towards this medical problem. One should not attempt to hide his allergies. At times this can be dangerous. If a person has allergies he should admit it and receive the best possible medical care available.

If persons in school situations, at summer camps, or places of employment are not informed about allergic problems it is possible for a sudden dangerous situation to arise. This could happen especially if someone were exquisitely allergic to stinging insects or to certain foods. Odours can sometimes cause sudden alarming symptoms. Persons in positions of authority at school and work should be aware of allergies and have appropriate treatment medication available for emergency use.

CHAPTER TWO

Nose and eye allergies

ALLERGIES AFFECTING THE NOSE

What is hay fever?

Hay fever is an allergy which affects either or both the eyes and the nose. If it affects only the nose it is called allergic rhinitis ("rhin" refers to the nose and "itis" refers to an inflammation). It is also sometimes called allergic rhinorrhea which means flowing or watery discharge from the nose. This problem affects up to 10 per cent of the population. It does not cause a fever and although hay can cause nose allergies, many other substances also can.

Some patients have year-round nose symptoms and this is called "perennial allergic rhinitis". If the nose symptoms are noted only during a particular time of the year or season when a certain pollen or substance is in the air, it is more correctly termed "seasonal allergic rhinitis" or "seasonal pollinosis". See pages 24 and 260.

What are the signs and symptoms of hay fever?

Patients who have this problem may have one or any combination of the following. The more of these a person has, the more severe the allergic problem is.

1. Watery nose mucus
2. Stuffiness, sniffling and "snorting". The stuffiness may or may not be associated with watery mucus.
3. Sneezing several times in a row, especially upon arising in the morning.
4. Breathing with an open mouth.
5. In some way wiggling the nose or wrinkling it. Some children massage the end of the nose with their palm or rub it upwards towards their forehead, or pick at their nose. The movement is usually not sideways. If they continually rub their nose upwards it causes a wrinkle to form across the bridge of the nose which is very characteristic of allergies and in adolescents it is frequently outlined with blackheads.
6. An itchy roof of the mouth, ear canals, or throat.

7. Throat-clearing.
8. Recurrent episodes of nose bleeding.
9. Circles under the eyes called "allergic shiners".
10. Puffy eyes – this refers to the skin below, above or along side the eyes. Adults can detect this problem in themselves. Mothers may notice a puffiness or unusual look about their youngster's eyes just prior to the onset of an allergic episode. It is sometimes possible to abort an allergic episode by immediately giving the allergy drugs if such a warning signal is noticed.
11. Inability to smell or taste. This will occur if the nose remains blocked from the swelling of the tissue or membranes lining the nose. This also frequently occurs when someone has a cold or upper respiratory infection and at that time would be unrelated to allergy.

How can you tell nose allergies from a cold?

Sometimes this is very easy. If a person has many of the signs and symptoms mentioned in the previous answer, the patient probably has allergies. When you look inside the nostrils with a flash light, notice if the tissue in the nose is paler than the lips. There should be no dry crusts in the nose and if mucus were present, it would be watery. At times, the inside of the nose is merely very swollen, pale and no mucus is evident. The only problem is stuffiness.

In contrast, if the tissues within the nose are much redder than the lips and there is thick, grey, green or yellow secretions or dried crusts, this would probably indicate infection. In addition when infection is evident, other members of the family or the person who has this problem may be ill and have a fever. Persons who have allergies affecting their nose are often irritable and fussy, but they are not sick.

It sometimes becomes difficult to tell the difference between allergy and infection when both are present at the same time. Many patients who have allergies are found to have a proneness towards infection but fortunately the latter problem often subsides after the allergies are treated and the nose tissues become more normal in appearance and size. It is sometimes confusing to tell an allergy from an early viral infection (upper respiratory infection or a cold) because both cause watery nose mucus. Later however mucus from virus infection becomes quite thick and cloudy grey.

Does hay fever alter a person's disposition?

Yes. Hay fever patients, children and adults, often become irritable, moody, listless, and unlike themselves. Children will cry for little reason and fuss more than normal. This problem subsides once they have received treatment for their allergies. Affected persons may not sleep as well if their nose is stuffed at night and so they are not well rested in the morning. Persons with hay fever are sometimes more subdued and quiet than normal and have difficulties in their coordination. These effects are often due to the use of antihistamines which can interfere with their work, school, or play. An attempt should be made to change the drug so that one is used which does not have this undesirable effect. Antihistamines which make children or adults sleepy should be only used at bedtime or not used at all.

When do people have hay fever?

Some patients have symptoms all year-round either every day or intermittently. Symptoms are often more severe in the morning and again at bedtime and tend to lessen in the middle of the day. Classical hay fever symptoms are seasonal in nature and caused by pollens or mould spores which are prevalent in the air at specific times. In each area of a country, different tree, grass, and weed pollens and mould spores are evident, each being in the air for one to several weeks. If a person is allergic to one of these, each year at about the same time, symptoms would recur unless the patient had been treated.

How are nose allergies treated.

1. If the problem is on and off throughout the year the initial treatment would be to try to determine whether it was caused by something in the house or a food. (See pages 137, 158). If the offending substance can be avoided or not eaten, nose allergies should diminish or disappear. Allergy injection treatments would be necessary if avoidance did not sufficiently relieve a patient's symptoms.

2. If the offending substances are pollens these can be diminished by using an electronic air filter within a patient's bedroom or home. Allergy injection therapy for pollens is often necessary to help patients who have this type of allergy.

3. It helps if the pollen sensitive patient can remain indoors rather than being outside, especially on windy days because pollen exposure inside a home is much less than that found outdoors.

4. Antihistamines (page 103) dry mucous secretions, decrease nose tissue swelling and help stop the itchy feeling in the nose. Sometimes nose allergic symptoms disappear shortly after arising in the morning and no antihistamines should or need be taken. Antihistamines should be used only if sneezing, stuffiness, watery mucus or nose discomfort interferes with normal activity, sleep, or tends to make a person uncomfortable.

5. Nose drops of various types can be helpful, especially for sudden or prolonged swelling within the nose. There are some types of nose drops which help for short periods of time and others which help for more prolonged periods. Some can be purchased without a prescription. Some

physicians do not recommend the use of nose drops because older children and adults overuse them. Normally nose drops can be used two or three times a day for approximately two or three days. If used for a longer period than three days, however, they may irritate the inside of the nostrils and cause the nose tissues to swell producing more stuffiness. At this point the tendency to use more nose drops occurs and a vicious cycle is begun. It is difficult to stop the use of nose drops once this happens and a physician's help may be necessary. (See page 105).

Nose drugs are most effective if used in the following way: Have the patient spray nose medicine into one nostril and wait five minutes. He should then blow his nose and spray again into the same nostril. This will shrink the upper portions of the nose passage-way and more effectively help breathing. The same procedure should be repeated in the other nostril. If nose drops are used the head should be tipped back as far as possible and the nose drops placed directly in the nostril. One or two drops should be used and in five minutes the nose should be blown so that the second application will help to shrink the upper nasal passages. Medicated ointments should not be placed within the nostrils. These may irritate the inside of the nose. If using nose drops in infants or children be certain that the type you use is safe. Some types of nose drops are too strong, except for adults.

6. Masks can be worn over the nose to prevent irritating substances from being breathed. These however are not always practical because many adults and children do not want to be seen wearing such a mask. They can be worn however when dusting or cleaning an area such as a garage or basement. These masks are of different types, and in general the more expensive ones are more efficient.

7. Occasionally if nose symptoms are very severe, a cortisone or special medicine in nose spray might be advised by your physician. These types should be used no longer than your doctor recommends.

8. Aspirin is often helpful in decreasing the effect of nose allergies. This can safely be used with antihistamines if this combination is effective. Aspirin should never be used by persons who are allergic to this drug. Certain aspirin substitutes are available which can safely be used.

What are common complications of nose allergies?
1. Recurrent infection can sometimes be a problem. The inside of the nose swells and the tissues become less resistant to infection because they are puffy and the blood supply is less than normal. Germs are within everyone's nose and can cause infection at any time. In children infections tend to spread to the ears and the throat while in adults and older children the sinuses are more often affected causing headaches located near the eyes. Chest infections can also be related to recurrent nose allergies.

There are some physicians who believe that it is helpful if a combination of nose drops and antihistamines are used *immediately* at the first sign of an infection. This is thought possibly to decrease the penetration of the infecting germs and possibly prevent or shorten the course of the infection.

2. Bronchial asthma is a possible complication of severe hay fever. Coughing, in excess, especially with exercise or emotional upsets such as laughter, or shortness of breath are often warnings that chest allergies are about to begin. It is possible but relatively uncommon for a hay fever patient to develop asthma after his hay fever has been treated. Allergy injection treatments in themselves usually do not cause asthma (except possibly as an immediate reaction if the dose is too large. (See page 127). When asthma occurs in a treated hay fever patient it is most often because he has developed a new allergy which affects the chest rather than the nose and eyes.

3. At times watery swellings called nose polyps develop within the nose of adults. Preadolescent children rarely have polyps. If they are noted they might signify either cystic fibrosis or chronic sinus infection. Patients with nose polyps and aspirin sensitivity often have severe, difficulty to control, asthma. (See page 210).

4. Patients who have nose allergies for long periods of time develop a characteristic facial appearance. They continually rub their nose upwards causing a horizontal crease or allergic nose wrinkle across the bridge of the nose. Because the nose tissue swells causing pressure on the blood vessels, the blood in the veins near the eyes and nose can't drain properly. This causes "allergic shiners" or dark circles under the eyes. Puffiness in the region of the eyes may be on a similar basis. Children who mouth breathe have relatively small noses and larger mouths. Dental deformities are also noted because of the long narrow palates in children who have nose allergies and these require orthodontal treatment.

5. Some nose allergic patients tend to have recurrent nose bleeds. Sometimes this is the sole or major manifestation of nose allergies. Most nose bleeds are caused by delicate superficial blood vessels which are located in the area which divides the two halves of the nose (nasal septum). These blood vessels sometimes have to be cauterized or burned so that the bleeding problem no longer occurs. Other nose bleeds are due to nose picking caused by dried mucus crusts within the nose. Your nose specialist or allergist could determine whether allergy, superficial blood vessels, or dried mucus is the cause of a nose bleed problem.

Can allergy cause a loss of ability to smell?
It can. This is sometimes noted in relation to food allergies or when a patient is having severe seasonal hay fever symptoms. Usually the sense

of smell will return once the substance causing the allergies is avoided or treatments have been received. Because other serious medical conditions can cause a loss of smell, you should be thoroughly examined by your physician if this problem is noted.

Adults who suffer from nose polyps often have no sense of smell and may also complain of a decrease in their sense of taste. A loss of smell can occur months and years before nasal polyps can be seen by the doctor.

What is non-allergic or vasomotor rhinitis?

Some patients have nose complaints or catarrh or a stuffed nose similar to persons having typical nose allergies. It is called vasomotor rhinitis. It is not caused by exposure to allergenic substances but rather triggered by chilling draughts, fatigue, tobacco smoke, odours, high humidity or emotional upsets, such as fright, anger, or excitement. Some can have sneezing and a profuse watery nasal mucus, associated with a complete loss of smell. Such patients may have negative allergy skin tests and have no eosinophils (See page 121) in their nose mucus. Antihistamines (pages 103-105), ephedrine-like drugs (page 106), and aspirin sometimes help non-allergic rhinitis. Attempt to decrease draughts, chilling, or exposure to odours, such as smoke. Nose specialists (otolaryngologists) may help by detecting and treating structure abnormalities in the nose which can contribute to this problem. Some patients have both nose allergies and vasomotor rhinitis.

What other non-allergic conditions cause nose symptoms?.

Some women have nose symptoms only during pregnancy. The relationship between having a baby and a runny nose seems to be due to hormones.

Persons with thyroid deficiencies can also have watery nose mucus and pale nose tissues. This type of nose problem stops after thyroid hormone treatment.

The excessive use of nose drops or sprays can cause nose blockage as discussed on page 105. If irritating nose preparations are stopped entirely, improvement can begin in about four days and the patient may be able to breathe normally in a week or two. The period of discomfort during the first few days after stopping nose drops can be decreased by using antihistamines or medicines prescribed by your physician.

Other problems which cause nose blockage are related to sinus infections or foreign objects, within the nose. A constant runny nose and sneezing, localized however to one nostril can be seen in patients who have a histamine-type headache. (See page 93).

How are sinuses related to allergic problems?

It is believed by some persons that the sinuses can *directly* be affected by allergies in much the same way as the lungs can be affected in persons who have asthma or the skin in patients who have eczema. The sinuses are holes or cavities within the bones located in the area of the nose. The sinus air cavities open through a passageway into the nose. This passageway allows air to enter the sinuses and mucus to pass out of the sinuses. Normally mucus is continually formed by glands within the sinuses and this mucus is moved by tiny hairs out of the sinuses, a process which keeps the sinus cavities clean. If the membranes lining the sinuses are directly affected by allergies, they can swell and cause more secretions to form than normal. If the swelling is extreme it can cause fluid to be trapped within the sinus cavity and this can create a sinus headache. Such headaches may be located above or below one or both eyes or between the eyes. The location of the headache would depend upon which sinus happened to be involved. If germs are trapped in the mucus in the sinus cavities, it causes a sinus infection. In these patients the mucus coming from the sinus areas would probably be green or yellow. Fever is usually but not always noticed when a patient has a sinus infection. Sinus problems are often *indirectly* caused by swelling of the tissues within the nose. The allergically swollen tissue can block normal drainage from the sinus cavities. Many adults have sinus problems but are unaware that their basic difficulty is not within the sinus but within the nose. Morning stuffiness, watery nasal secretions, sneezing in series, and itching within the nose would all indicate nose allergies and if these symptoms were associated with sinus problems, by treating the nose allergies, the sinus problems might stop. Other common problems which contribute to sinus disease would be enlarged adenoids, deformities or abnormalities in the structure of the nose, or diseased teeth.

If a person's sinus problems are related to nose allergies the use of an antihistamine and nose drops might help temporarily. These help shrink the swollen tissues within the nose so that proper drainage from the sinuses could occur. If infection is present, antibiotics might have to be prescribed by your physician. The application of heat to the face in the region of the sinuses is sometimes helpful because this thins the sinus mucus so that it could drain more readily. Special heating pads to help concentrate heat over the sinus areas are sometimes available. If sinus problems are due to allergies, the best treatment is to determine what is causing the swelling within the nose so that this problem could be eliminated.

ALLERGIES AFFECTING THE EYES

Which symptoms are typical of eye allergy?
Itchiness of the eyes, reddening of the white portion (the conjunctiva)

and tearing are characteristic. Rarely, only one eye is affected if an allergenic substance touches only one eye. For example most people tend to rub an itchy eye and if cat dandruff (dander) is on the fingers the condition quickly becomes worse. The white part of the eye can swell enormously so that the eye seems to be filled with jelly. Typical causes of eye allergies are pollen, mould spores, animals, foods, or dust.

Patients who have eczema or skin allergies frequently have dry upper eyelids and it is important to try to determine whether the skin near the eye or surface of eyeball is itching. Certain contact skin disease caused by fingernail polish, eye cosmetics, shampoos, or hair preparations can affect the upper eyelid skin.

Because there are many eye problems which can cause similar symptoms, a physician should definitely be consulted.

What indicates infection of the eye?

Yellow or discoloured mucus on the surface of the eye or eyelashes could indicate infection. This is frequently a complication of eye allergies unless the hands are kept very clean.

How can eye allergic symptoms be relieved?

1. Cleanse the surface of the eyeball by merely opening the eyes under water. Children will readily do this in a clean bathtub or bowl of water. Adults use an eye cleansing solution and an eye cup. The eye wash should be at room temperature or very slightly warmed so that it does not irritate the eye. One blinks the eye while the eye cup containing the eye wash is in place. Be certain to boil the eye cup between use if infection is present in the eye.

2. There are special eye drops which contain ephedrine to diminish itching. Eye drops can be easily applied if a person's head is tipped backwards and a couple of drops are placed on the little pink mound on the inner corner of the eye. Be careful not to touch the eye while doing this so the eye solution is not contaminated. Pull the lower eyelid downwards and the drop will fall from the pink rounded spot to the area between the lower eyeball and lowered eyelid. This causes blinking which spreads the medicine over the outer surface of the eye.

3 Because allergenic substances blow in the eye it helps if curved, large sunglasses protect the eye. Glasses help when riding in a car near an open window or on a motorcycle or bicycle.

4 Antihistamines help diminish itching and swelling of eye allergies. (See page 103).

5. The hands should be washed frequently to reduce the possibility of introducing germs into the eyes when they are rubbed.

6. Cortisone eye drops are available from your physician if the above do not effectively eliminate the eye symptoms.

Can the white portion become very swollen from allergies?

At times the white part of the eye can bulge and swell beyond the eyelids. Your allergist or eye physician should be contacted although the measures described previously might help temporarily.

Is it dangerous for the eye to swell completely closed?

Extreme eye swelling will not usually permanently damage the eye or the skin around the eyes although a person's face could temporarily have a most distorted appearance. Insect stings on the face or even mosquito bites sometimes cause marked swelling. If infection contributes to excessive eye swelling, the lids are frequently stuck together with discoloured mucus. A physician should therefore examine the eyes to determine the exact cause and treatment of this condition.

What other form of eye allergy is sometimes a problem?

A rare form of eye allergy is vernal conjunctivitis. This commonly is present in the late spring and early summer and tends to persist through the warm weather season, or sometimes throughout the year. It seldom occurs before the age of ten years and rarely after the age of 30. It often disappears after approximately 5 to 15 years. Most patients who have this problem have obvious allergies or allergies within their family. In addition to a cobblestone appearance of the inner eyelids, there is redness, burning, and itching of both eyes and increased tear formation. A ropey discharge causes intense irritation and must be carefully removed. Your doctor can examine the mucus to determine if it contains a certain type of white blood cell which is characteristic of allergies and called an eosinophil.

No one knows exactly what causes this eye problem. It is aggravated by exposure to light and heat. If pollen hayfever makes the condition worse, allergy injection therapy would be indicated. It is a particularly severe problem in persons living in desert areas because of associated irritation from sand and the prevalence of trachoma infections.

This disease is difficult to treat and the services of an eye specialist are always required. Cortisone drops are often necessary to help relieve the condition.

CHAPTER THREE

Chest allergies

COUGHS DUE TO ALLERGIES

What is characteristic about an allergic cough?

An allergic cough often is diagnosed because it does not respond to cough syrups or antibiotic treatment. Chest allergies can cause an excessive cough for days, weeks or even years before the first wheezing episode or may never cause wheezing. Quite often people who are coughing do not know they are also wheezing.

An allergic cough is caused by slight spasm of the air tubes or an excessive amount of lung mucus. This cough surprisingly does not always respond to the type of drugs used to treat asthma. Patients who have this problem may notice that it is worse during exercise or when there is an emotional upset such as laughter, anger, or excitement. This cough may disappear completely when a patient's home is made allergy-free, a food which is causing allergies is eliminated, or when allergy extract therapy is received. (See Chapters 10, 11, 12).

Is there a way to tell the difference between various types of coughs?

There are many factors which cause coughing. Three major common causes are sometimes relatively easy to tell apart.

1. The first type of cough is due to a tickle in the throat noted when a person has an infection. This cough may be helped by a cough syrup or by treatment with an antibiotic. If a person has an infection it is usually obvious because he feels unwell. He has a cold, sore thoat, fever, or green or yellow mucus. The cough is often deep, hoarse, and sometimes sounds like a puppy's bark.

2. In contrast to an infection-type cough there is another due to a postnasal drip of mucus. This often causes "throat-clearing". Most affected persons are aware that their nose mucus is dripping down the back of their throat. This cough is generally worse at night and can cause children to make a "clucking" sound. It becomes less severe with exercise because the nose tends to clear with activity. As soon as the exertion is discontinued, however, the nose stuffs up and the cough recurs.

31

Antihistamines often help.

3. The cough which precedes or is associated with wheezing is almost always made worse by exertion or exercise, or by an emotional upset, either happy or sad. This type of cough is sometimes helped by a medicine which is used to treat asthma or one which contains an ephedrine-like drug (Salbutamol or Terbutaline).

Are allergic coughs always associated with asthma?

No. It is possible to have a cough as the sole manifestation of chest allergy, although it may precede wheezing by minutes, months or years. Some patients notice the cough is entirely eliminated after they receive their allergy injection treatments (See Chapter 10) and just before they need a booster treatment they will notice that the cough recurs. The best treatment for this is to receive the booster allergy extract treatments more often.

Adults and children may cough and not realize they are wheezing. Sometimes young children can tell when they are wheezing whereas older children and adults are unaware that there is spasm in their lungs. There is a marked variation regarding an individual's ability to detect if he is wheezing

All about Asthma

DIAGNOSIS, PROGNOSIS, TYPICAL CHARACTERISTICS, AND COMPLICATIONS

What is asthma?

Basically asthma means there is wheezing or a whistling sound when air is breathed from the lungs. Wheezing, however, can be caused by many medical problems other than allergy. In adults approximately one-half of asthmatic problems are not due to typical allergies. In children older than two years, wheezing is generally due to allergy. Allergies in the lungs cause swelling of the lining of the air tubes and spasm or tightening of the muscles around the air passages. This diminishes the size of the air tubes so that air whistles and squeaks as a person breathes out. If asthma is severe, the decrease in the size of the air tubes is so severe that there is also wheezing when air is breathed in. In addition, wheezing causes more mucus than normal to form within the lungs and this mucus can partially block the air passages. Infections, at any age also cause swelling of the inside of the air tubes and can, therefore, mimic allergic asthma. If you listen to someone's lungs it is not easy to tell whether it is the mucus of asthma or pus from infection which is heard. Bubbling or wet sounds are normally not heard in a well person's lungs.

What are the two main common types of asthma?

1. "Extrinsic" Asthma is caused primarily by known allergenic substances, such as dust, foods, pets, pollen, and moulds. (See page 39). The term extrinsic implies that it is caused by something *outside* of the body. This type causes most children's allergic asthma and about 50% of adult asthma.

2a. "Intrinsic" Asthma occurs much more frequently in adults. It is much less well-understood because the attacks are frequently associated with infection and irritants such as smoke. Patients who have intrinsic asthma tend to progress to chronic bronchitis and chronic lung infection. It frequently does not begin until middle age. The term intrinsic implies that the asthma is related to a problem *inside* the body.

2b. One variant of this type is discussed on page 26. It is associated with aspirin sensitivity and nose polyps. This type is often extremely difficult to treat.

How early in life can asthma occur?

It can begin very early in infancy. It often starts when a baby has a lung infection, pneumonia, whooping cough, flu, or after measles. Very young asthmatic children often have had a problem called bronchiolitis as an infant.

During the first year of life, allergic infants may have skin allergies, months of colic and "constant colds", which are not infections, but allergy. These problems may precede the first asthma attack. Asthma is seldom noted very early in infancy except in extremely allergic children. It more often occurs for the first time during childhood.

Can asthma first occur in middle life or later?

Yes. Asthma can occur at any age in a person's life. It is sometimes more difficult to treat when it first begins later in life. It is often associated with infection or due to unknown causes.

Is asthma more frequent in either sex?

For some unknown reason asthma occurs more frequently in boys than it does in girls, prior to puberty. This is also true of several other types of allergies. Hay fever is more common in males than females all over the world. This may be because men spend more time out of doors than women, exposing themselves to more pollen. A housewife who has seasonal pollen asthma may find it easier to stay indoors and thereby relieve her symptoms. Asthma occurring after the age of 40 in women seems to begin commonly when they notice change of life. During pregnancy about one-third of women are dramatically free of asthma, another third are worse and in the remaining third the asthma is not affected in anyway.

What causes allergic asthma?

As with other forms of allergies, the causes are often similar. Wheezing can occur for one to several weeks at a particular season of the year because of tree, grass, or weed pollens, or mould spores. (See page 3 for more details and page 260 for the pollination times in the area where you live.)

Year round wheezing occurs intermittently or every day, at any time during the year. This is often due to house dust (mites in the dust), furniture stuffing (kapok, cotton, animal hair, or wool), feathers, pet hair or dandruff, woollen carpets, perfumed substances, mould spores (in damp, wet, musty homes) and foods. (See pages 3 and 4, Chapter 1, Chapter 2 and Chapter 12).

Some patients have a combined type of allergy with intermittent or daily asthma throughout the year which is worse during the pollen season.

Infections often precipitate wheezing at any age and these are most evident during the colder months. Emotional upsets, fatigue, irritating odours, exercise or exertion, and infection often trigger asthmatic episodes. A combination of these factors may be related to the first episode of wheezing. This does not mean that these cause asthma, but they can trigger allergic problems. (See pages 2 and 5).

Smoke of all kinds is an irritant to everyone, especially the allergic patient. Cigarette smoke in a home, at work, and in a restaurant or automobile can cause the eyes to run, the nose to block, and the chest to wheeze. NO asthmatic should smoke and no parent should smoke in the presence of his allergic child.

How can you tell if someone is wheezing

It is not always easy to detect wheezing. Open your mouth and breathe deeply in and out so that there is no noise except for the sound of air passing in and out. It is important not to make any sound in your throat as you breathe. The sound you hear is coming from the lungs and this same sound is what you hear when you listen to a normal person breathing. If you want to examine a child, place your ear next to the naked chest or back and ask the youngster to take similar (quiet) very deep breaths in and out through the mouth. It helps if the nose is pinched so that nose sounds are not confused with lung sounds. If you hear a rattle, whistle or squeak as the person breathes, especially at the end of breathing out or exhaling, it could indicate a blockage to breathing such as a wheeze could cause. Allergic wheezing usually affects both lungs. If wheezing sounds are repeatedly heard only on one side, it could indicate a foreign object or obstruction is present within that lung and this individual should be checked thoroughly by a physician.

Some people can detect wheezing sounds easily in others or in themselves. Others are not able to do this. It might help if you ask your physician to allow you to listen with his stethoscope so that you can hear typical wheezing sounds. If wheezing is severe, it is easy to diagnose by most persons who have heard it before.

Sometimes children and adults do not wheeze unless they have laughed hard or exerted themselves. Have a person who might wheeze run about for a while and then listen to his lungs and see if the breath sounds remain clear. Wheezing may be heard only after someone has exercised and not when he is quiet and resting. This might be true especially if the person had not wheezed often or very much.

If a person is wheezing badly one does not have to be near to know that this is a problem. The whistling and squeaking sounds can be heard across the room. People may falsely believe that wheezing is present because they hear squeaks and whistling as they breathe. This can be caused from breathing through a partially plugged nose and may be completely unrelated to chest allergies. A whistling sound heard when someone is breathing, may be coming from the nose or the chest. You must try to learn the difference between a nose and chest whistle.

Sometimes no wheeze is present because there is so much difficulty in getting the air in and out of the lungs. Each breath can only take in half of the normal amount of air. Such patients become very breathless and wheezy with the slightest exertion.

Can a child outgrow asthma?

Yes, this is certainly possible. Some children wheeze a little with an infection. This occurs rarely and is never much of a problem. Many children, however, are allowed to wheeze for many years. The children and their parents have the incorrect impression that this problem will magically disappear as they age. During childhood, the youngster is unable to run, play, go to school, or carry on normal activities. If wheezing interferes with the youngster's normal way of life or if the problem seems to be recurrent and becoming more frequent or severe, an allergist should be consulted. It is amazing how often a youngster who cannot sleep at night and who wheezes every day will respond quickly and improve in a few days or weeks after his home has been made allergy-free or after he has been placed on a diet eliminating allergenic foods. Many patients improve from allergy extract therapy but it often requires several months. There are studies which indicate that boys sometimes improve spontaneously at puberty.

If an allergic problem receives proper management initially, asthma is much less apt to become a recurrent problem and a child should have a much better and more normal childhood. The chance of having chest problems during adult life should be less.

Some children or young adults grow out of asthma attacks but may find with strenuous exercise, they become a little wheezy. Twenty and thirty years later, they may develop asthma, which is quite severe, after years of freedom. This late recurrence of asthma may not be due to typical allergic causes, i.e., foods or substances within the home or in the outside air.

What percentage of asthmatics improve on therapy?

Children seem to respond more completely and better to proper and complete allergy treatment than adults. Part of this, as mentioned before, is due to the fact children's asthma is often due to an allergic problem whereas in adults many non-allergic factors need to be considered. When patients improve, their attacks become less severe and less frequent. Children may stop wheezing after several months of some combination of environmental control, dietary management, or allergy extract therapy. Some patients, maybe up to 10 per cent, will not respond as well as desired. These patients often require vigorous, constant, lifetime supervision and medication to handle acute wheezing episodes and to allow them to work and enjoy life as much as possible.

Does treated asthma stop and never recur?

It would be unusual for asthma to stop suddenly, and never to occur again. Attacks become less frequent and less severe when individuals improve. A patient may not have an attack for several years and suddenly because of an unfortunate set of circumstances begin to wheeze. This could happen if someone developed an infection at a time when he was fatigued or tired or when there was much excitement, such as during a holiday.

Parents become discouraged if a child has not wheezed for a long time and suddenly has a severe episode. They are fearful that the original problem has recurred. Persons who have asthma should try to look at the overall picture. How severe has the asthma been during a year or a period of several months? The attacks should be less prolonged and severe. Gradual, steady improvement is the allergist's aim and would indicate that the problem was certainly under control.

How should an episode of asthma be treated?

The best method to control asthma is to prevent it before it happens and this means avoiding known causes of allergies such as dust and pets. At times, however, this is not realistically possible. Adequate allergy extract therapy certainly eventually helps to decrease the number and intensity of many patients' asthmatic episodes, but until that time, parents or patients need to know what to do to help themselves until they can secure a physician's help.

The following suggestions are recommended:
1. During severe attacks, the person who is wheezing should stay in his allergy-free bedroom as much of the time as possible. Fluids should be given often to help keep the mucus thin so that it can be coughed up more readily. A general rule is a full glass of liquid every hour when the patient is awake. This liquid can be water, soft drinks or carbonated beverages, soup, tea, coffee, gelatin or iced desserts. The patient must be careful not to drink something which makes his asthma worse. Cola, chocolate, or cold liquids or foods adversely affect some patients.

2. The drugs used to treat asthma should be started at the *very first sign* of wheezing. Parents may notice a puffy look around their youngster's eyes or a certain type of cough or throat-clearing which serves as a warning that asthma is about to begin. If something indicates asthma, treatment should not be delayed. Repeated attacks may, however, become increasingly difficult to treat and if some of these episodes can be prevented by early treatment, this should be done. Some asthmatics delay using drugs so the physician can see how ill they are. It is felt that the doctor may know more about their problems if he can hear their wheezing. This should never be done. In general, the sooner an asthmatic episode is brought under control, the less severe it will be and less long it will last. Asthma should be considered a very bad habit and prevented whenever possible.

3. Asthma drugs are similar to a gallon of petrol. Treatment does not last forever. The fact that a drug helps for a few hours indicates that it is the correct one but it may need to be taken at regular intervals. It may take up to one-half hour before asthma drugs start to help and the effect will last 4 to possibly 12 hours. An asthma drug should be given according to schedule. Do not allow the lungs to go back into spasm because a dose of medicine is overdue. It is similar to driving your automobile. You do not allow the tank to become empty. You put in more petrol. When you are using asthma drugs, they help only so long and more should be taken before the effect of the previous dose is completely gone. Short-acting drugs (4 to 6 hours) are best for daytime use. Long-acting drugs (8 to 12 hours) should be used at bedtime. A long-acting medicine at bedtime would give more assurance of a full night's sleep than a short-acting one.

Patients who repeatedly forget to take their drugs at the proper time, will find their attacks are more difficult to control because they are allowing the air tubes repeatedly to go into spasm. This can greatly prolong the duration of an asthmatic attack.

4. Patients often have difficulty telling when they can stop using the asthma drugs. Drugs should be given as long as your physician specifies. If there is a question, check with him. Often when asthma is no longer obvious, i.e., no wheezes are heard when someone listens to that person's

chest, for 24 hours, the asthma drugs can be tapered . The middle of the day asthma dose is discontinued first, and if the patient is well, the morning dose then can be stopped. The night drug should be discontinued last because this is the time when most people wheeze. Don't be so cautious that you never stop the drugs. This is as erroneous as not giving treatment when an attack begins because you fear that you might become dependent upon pills.

There are a few other recommendations concerning the discontinuation of drugs. Many parents are afraid to taper medicines when a youngster has to go to school, so attempt to do this on weekends. If it is too soon to decrease a medicine, it can quickly be given, without any fear or concern. If a youngster's medicines are stopped while a child is attending school, check with the teacher or school nurse. It is surprisingly possible for some teachers with large classes to be so busy that they are not aware that a child is having severe respiratory problems. Children sometimes arrive home seriously ill because no one noticed and the child, for multiple reasons, did not call attention to the asthma.

What should you do if asthma recurs whenever drugs are stopped?

If this happens it means that whatever is causing the asthma is still present. Restart the asthma drugs at the dosage and interval recommended by your doctor. Attempt to try to find out why drugs continue to be needed. A physician's examination might reveal a hidden infection. Be sure the bedroom is allergy-free and no offending foods are being eaten. If a person needs daily asthma drugs this indicates he needs a physician's care. Check to be certain that the allergy extract is received at the proper dosage and frequency. (See pages 122-136)

How can middle of the night asthma be prevented and treated?

To prevent night attacks, take long-acting 8 to 12 hour medicines at bedtime rather than those which last only 4 to 6 hours. Early morning asthma attacks in children can often be prevented by giving the long-acting medicine at the parent's rather than the child's bedtime. This is helpful only if breathing problems do not occur when the child awakens.

Asthma sometimes suddenly occurs during sleep. Such attacks may be aborted if they are treated quickly. An inhaler is sometimes helpful. (See page 107).

Should a wheezing youngster be sent to school?

The answer to this question depends upon a doctor's and parent's philosophy. If the wheezing was mild and easily controlled by medicine, the youngster could probably be sent to school. For example, if a child wheezed from playing with a neighbour's cat but slept well during the night, the mother might send her youngster to school after giving asthma medicine. If, however, the youngster was possibly beginning an infection, even though the asthma was mild, it would be better to keep the youngster home so that he could be observed and seen by a physician if necessary.

Infection often causes a fever, sore throat, pain, an abdominal upset, or green or yellow mucus, but this is certainly not true in all children. Many times they can be sick and there is no obvious sign of infection. If there is any question about infection, a physician's examination should reveal the diagnosis and best treatment. Different infections are treated for shorter and longer periods of time and these questions cannot be answered except after a physical examination.

If a youngster is in obvious distress or has had a difficult night, he should definitely *not* be sent to school. Permissive parents have difficulty in this regard because their children say they are well and want to go to school because there is a test or a party. In this situation mature adult judgment is required and permissiveness cannot be tolerated. If the mother needs re-assurance, or if she is unsure of what to do, she should check with the doctor.

One other problem is that some children don't want to go to school and they use their illness as a crutch. Parents must use mature judgment. If their child looks well and had a good night he should be sent to school.

One frequent problem is that a mother who works or has certain commitments on a particular day, may tend to send her youngster to school too soon. The decision should not be what is most convenient but what is best for the child. A babysitter may have to be secured. The final consideration must be only what is best for your child's health.

When should you contact your doctor about an asthma attack?

If the attack is severe and you are concerned, contact your doctor. If the proper drugs have been given but the asthma is not improving, contact your doctor. If the wheezing is slight or moderately severe, day after day in spite of treatment, check with your physician. Most asthmatic episodes tend to clear up in a matter of hours or a day or two.

How can you tell what causes an asthma attack?

Many patients seldom wheeze. If a person is alert and spends a few minutes thinking about why an episode occurs, it may be possible to determine the cause and prevent future episodes. A mother can often tell from the way her child acts or looks that an attack is about to begin. She should immediately think about what was different than usual. Why did the attack occur today and not yesterday, this afternoon and not this morning? The cause could be infection (fever, sore throat, congestion, intestinal upset, or green or yellow mucus) especially if other members of the family are sick.

If someone always wheezes when an infection starts, give asthma drugs immediately and contact your physician. Sometimes asthmatic episodes can be aborted by using asthma drugs and antibiotics as soon as possible.

Other common causes of sudden asthma attacks are visiting someone's home, painting or remodelling, cleaning dusty or damp areas, contact with pets, or exposure to anything which is new or different.

One should also consider drugs. Aspirin taken for an infection may cause wheezing. It is easy to incorrectly assume that the infection caused the asthma attack, when in fact, it was aspirin.

Foods or pets sometimes cause wheezing only during a pollen season. Melons and bananas may cause symptoms *only* when eaten during the weed season but not during the remainder of the year. Pet allergies which occur only during pollen seasons can sometimes be due to hair or dandruff (See page 191), but also can be caused by pollen on the animal's fur after walking through grass or weeds.

How can you count someone's respirations?

In order to count someone's breathing rate, you need a watch which has a second hand. Count the number of times that the person breathes in and out for one full minute. Count an entire breath in-*and*-out, as only one.

The rate of breathing can be easily counted across the room if asthma is severe. The "in-and-out" breaths can easily be heard.

For slight asthma, watch the chest or abdomen to count the breathing rate. Count one for each time the abdomen goes up *and* down or the skin between the ribs moves in *and* out. It is impossible to count a breathing rate during crying, laughter or talking. Do not try to count the respiratory rate for 15 seconds and multiply by 4, unless you are experienced. It would be better to count for a minute or two.

Why is the respiratory rate important?

It helps to tell whether wheezing is becoming better or worse. If the attack is becoming more severe, the number of times a patient breathes each minute will increase. If a patient is "holding his own", the respiratory rate will stay about the same. After a patient starts to improve the breathing rate decreases. The night respiratory rate should be less than the day rate. It helps a doctor if you report the breathing rate was 20 this morning and is now 50 per minute.

On occasion a patient may look sicker even though the respiratory rate is not increasing. If you are concerned, check with the doctor.

How fast should someone breathe?

An infant normally breathes at about 30 or 40 times a minute, children at 20 to 25 and adults at a rate of 16 to 20 per minute. If a breathing rate is consistently over 50 in a youngster, a physician should be notified. If the rate is continually increasing or the patient seems worse, contact a physician or go to the nearest hospital.

How can you tell when asthma is worse or better?
When a person has severe asthma, he does not talk, smile or eat, although he may drink fluids. He will be unable to sleep. (Do not give drugs which cause sleep) Trying to breath is a full time occupation.
When a patient starts to improve, the first evidence is often hunger. He will begin to smile, talk, and is able to lie flat. A sure sign of improvement is the ability of an exhausted patient to sleep.

Is it important if an asthmatic's face turns white?
This may not be a bad sign. Adrenaline frequently makes a patient look pale. Prolonged wheezing can cause a white face, cold and clammy skin, and somewhat blue fingernails and lips. A physician should be notified if this occurs.

Does asthma cause excess perspiration?
When children and adults wheeze, they may perspire so heavily that their hair is wet. This stops once the attack is over. Some persons, especially males, normally perspire in excess.

How important are blue lips or fingernails?
This is not a good sign. It means that there is not enough oxygen in the blood. Contact your physician.
Young children frequently have blue lips when they swim in cold water, especially if they are chilled or fatigued. This responds to rest and warmth and is entirely unrelated to asthma.

Is it possible to wheeze and not know it?
It certainly is. Sometimes a young child can detect the slightest asthma while an adult can't. There is a marked individual difference in the ability of people to know when they wheeze. Patients can better detect wheezing by breathing very deeply in *and* out. A wheeze may be noticeable *only* at the end of a deep breath.

Are asthma drugs needed when someone is *not* wheezing?
There are four situations when someone who is *not* wheezing should take asthma drugs to prevent asthma.
1. One common cause of asthma is exertion or exercise. Drugs to stop asthma should be taken 20 minutes prior to any activity known to cause wheezing. Children may always wheeze when they take gym or ride their

bikes. Medicine before play allows children and adults to exercise.

2. Another common cause of asthmatic episodes are happy or sad emotional situations. An adult may find that he often wheezes at work or home if something unpleasant happens. If a youngster is upset at school or home, medicines to help asthma should be given to prevent a wheezing episode. Hearty laughter or the excitement of holidays, trips, or birthdays can precipitate asthma, especially if someone is fatigued or tired. Use asthma drugs prophylactically for these situations.

If reprimands cause asthma, a youngster should be medicated if possible 10 minutes before he's disciplined. If this is not done, you may have a spoiled child and behaviour problems in the other children. Once the allergies have responded to treatment, prophylactic medicines may not be necessary.

3. Some individuals wheeze with every infection. If asthma drugs are given at the first sign of infection along with drugs for the infection, the asthma attack may be prevented or aborted.

4. One infrequent cause of asthma noted in females seems to be related to their menstrual cycle or pregnancy. Some women wheeze prior to each menses or throughout each pregnancy. Why this happens is not understood but asthma drugs should be taken if they prevent these episodes. Check with your allergist and your obstetrician concerning the safety of any drug taken during pregnancy.

Is it important to drink fluids when wheezing?

During an asthma attack, there is an increased amount of mucus in the lungs. If this mucus becomes too thick and sticky, it is difficult to cough up. Mucus causes it to become progressively more difficult to breathe. It is essential that fluids in large amounts be taken so the thick mucus can be more easily coughed up. During severe asthma a patient may not eat, but he absolutely must drink. At least one glass should be taken every hour when the patient is awake. Do not awaken sleeping asthmatics to give them liquids because the motion of sitting up can cause coughing and subsequent wheezing. When a patient awakens at night and takes drugs, he should drink a large quantity of water. If sufficient fluids are not taken, severe asthma may necessitate hospitalization so that intravenous fluids can be given. Liquids are also necessary to help replace the large amounts of body moisture lost during asthmatic breathing.

If a patient can't cough up mucus, special medicines may be needed to help thin the mucus. Spitting does not normally occur until about the age of 7 years. Young children tend to cough up but not spit out mucus. Instead they swallow it and sometimes this accumulation in their stomach causes a bellyache. If the mucus is vomited from the stomach, it should be examined. If it is green or yellow, it could indicate infection and your physician should be notified.

It is difficult to tell if sufficient fluids have been taken. If the tongue looks dry or sticks to the inside of the mouth, the patient needs more fluids.

Which fluids are best during asthma?

Any liquid is helpful except those which obviously worsen asthma. Patients may be given soup, tea, warm beverages of various types, or diluted gelatin before it has set. If cold liquids do not adversely affect the patient, ice cream, iced forms of dessert, or gelatin can be taken. Persons allergic to chocolate or cocoa should not drink cola beverages because these could worsen asthma.

Which methods help to remove mucus from the lungs?

By positioning the body properly, mucus can more readily be cleared from the lungs. These methods are part of pulmonary physiotherapy and can be taught by trained persons in large hospitals. Massaging and pounding the back helps move mucus from certain sectors of the lungs. If a physiotherapist knows which lung sectors are badly affected, specific exercises can be done to drain that particular area.

Mucus drainage is more effective if attempts are made to open the air tubes more fully by using asthma drugs before therapy exercise. Try also to thin lung mucus so that it is easier to expel by drinking large amounts of fluid each day and using special drugs prescribed by your physician.

Can "cold" cause allergic coughing or asthma?

Cold air or cold liquids or foods can sometimes cause immediate asthma. Once patients, however, are well-treated they may be able to drink refrigerated cold liquids whereas this might not have been possible previously. If a person has difficulty in the cold outside air, he should breathe through his nose, not his mouth. The nose passageway tends to warm air so it is not as cold when it reaches the lungs. It might also help if the nose and mouth were covered by a non-allergic scarf in very cold weather.

Does wheezing cause vomiting?

It often does, especially in children under the age of 7 years. The excessive lung mucus is coughed up and swallowed causing abdominal discomfort.

Tiny hairs called cilia line the lung tubes and carry mucus to the back of the throat where it is normally swallowed or spit out. This mucus movement occurs constantly and helps to keep the lungs clear of foreign particles. Movement is decreased in persons who smoke tobacco but exaggerated in asthmatics because there is more mucus to move.

If a person vomits, he expels mucus and stomach contents but in addition he brings up mucus from the lungs. For this reason, vomiting may sometimes help relieve asthma temporarily. Always check the colour of the mucus. Cloudy white or colourless is probably normal but green or yellow could indicate infection which your physician would want to treat.

Asthma often causes an upset stomach. If a wheezing child travels in an automobile, always carry a paper bag or container just in case he vomits.

Is vomiting ever a serious problem for an asthmatic?
Yes, it can be. Extreme vomiting can cause an excessive loss of fluid from the body. This combined with the fluid loss from the lungs during rapid breathing can cause many problems which require a physician's help. A medicine called theophylline (See page 107) is often used to treat asthma. It can cause vomiting of a coffee ground-like material if it is taken in too large a dose.

If a patient is vomiting all drugs, asthma can be controlled by rectal or injected medicines. If a patient has *both* vomiting and diarrhoea, medicines can't be taken by mouth or rectum. Asthma drugs would have to be given by injection and hospitalization might be required. The exact cause of vomiting must also be diagnosed so it can be treated.

What helps an upset belly when someone wheezes?
This is often relieved if the patient vomits. This can be induced by putting a finger down the throat. In young children, care must be taken so that they do not choke and get vomited material into their lungs.

The discomfort may be helped if heat (a hot water bottle or a heating pad) is applied to the abdomen. Cola drinks sometimes settle the stomach (providing the patient is not allergic to chocolate). The carbonated gas can be eliminated by adding sugar or allowing an uncapped bottle of cola to sit at room temperature.

If abdominal discomfort seems prolonged or severe, a physician should be notified. For example, if a patient has received large doses of cortisone (See page 112) for a prolonged period of time, a stomach ulcer could develop which may cause pain.

What common complications of asthma can occur?
1. The most frequent is bronchitis or pneumonia (See page 47). These usually respond well and quickly to the appropriate antibiotic. Most patients will have a temperature and green or yellow mucus, in addition to excessive coughing. Patients who have pneumonia frequently cough more than they wheeze. Such patients may also have very active nostril movements when they breath. This, however, can also occur with severe asthma. The outer portion of the nostrils do not actively move when

someone has mild wheezing.

Asthma drugs alone will not control wheezing unless any associated infection is also properly treated. An antibiotic is often necessary, although viral infections would not be helped by antibiotics.

2. The lung is similar to a mass of connected tiny ballons which all eventually open into the windpipe. Occasionally if a person coughs or wheezes very hard a bubble forms on the outside of one of the balloons and if this breaks, certain lung sectors near that area would collapse because air leaks out. If a significant portion of someone's lung collapses it can cause sudden extreme chest pain, marked breathing difficulty and blue lips and fingernails. This is called a pneumothorax and if there is a possibility that this has happened, contact your physician or go to the nearest hospital. It is not unusual for someone's chest to ache or hurt from wheezing severely for a long time but sudden very severe chest pain indicates that a physician is needed.

3. On occasion wheezing causes the lung to develop a slow leak similar to that seen in a tyre. The leak is tiny so that the lung does not really collapse but air can escape and move into the upper chest near the lower neck. When touched, this area feels as if there are little movable bubbles under the skin. If the skin in the region of the neck and collarbone feels different from the rest of the body, a physician should be consulted.

4. When someone wheezes badly, the lungs fill with a larger amount of mucus than normal. This mucus often becomes very thick, especially if adequate fluids are not taken. On occasion this mucus becomes so thick that it plugs some of the lung's air passages. If this happens, a lung sector collapses because air cannot pass through a mucus plug. This is called atelectasis. This sort of problem can cause great difficulty breathing and often requires a physician.

5. It is easier for an asthmatic to get air into the lungs than it is to get it out. This can lead to overdistended lungs and temporary or permanent changes in the size and shape of the chest. These factors can contribute to the development of emphysema. (See page 59).

What personal attitudes help asthma?

You should realize that your asthma drugs should control most episodes. If the drugs are not helping well enough or fast enough, check with the doctor. Undue anxiety intensifies breathing problems. Have faith in your drugs and doctor. Try to relax.

Parents or relatives who look frightened, or act flustered can make someone's asthma worse. Parents do not have to express concern in words. A child can tell if his parent's upset by looking at his face. If a parent looks calm and confident, this in itself will relax a child and aid his breathing. For example, many patients feel better as soon as they walk into the doctor's office or as soon as the physician enters the room. This is because they feel they are about to be helped. Parents, spouses or relatives can convey similar confidence and assurance if they do not appear frightened. If someone can't mask his feelings he should avoid caring for someone during an asthma attack.

When does severe asthma require a physician?

This is difficult to answer but if breathing causes extreme distress or gasping for breath, your physician should be called. The appropriate drugs should be given immediately and the correct treatment should obviously help in 20 or 30 minutes. Some severe asthmatic episodes cause the notches in the lower central neck and above the collarbones to be sucked in, as well as the areas between the ribs. This indicates a severe struggle to breathe. If a patient can eat, talk, smile, make jokes and sleep, the asthma is not severe. If a patient is spending all of his energy breathing and is paying little attention to anything else, he is quite ill.

During an asthma attack, the face may appear anxious and a patient will sit so he is hunched forward. The neck appears to be pulled in because the shoulders are raised and the hands may be braced against his knees. Breathing may be very noisy during both inspiration and expiration. Occasionally someone may have extreme difficulty breathing but makes no noise because he can't move air either in or out of the lungs. Severe asthma causes a pale and moist face and blue lips. Very severe sudden chest pain indicates a physician is needed. (See page 41).

The muscular exertion involved in wheezing or coughing for long periods of time can make the chest ache. Adults and particularly pregnant women may break a rib during a severe cough. The fracture may be heard by the patient and causes localized pain with each breath for the next week or so.

Can a person die from asthma?

Fortunately, this seldom occurs, but it certainly can happen. Asthma is a common complaint, death from it is uncommon. If someone has severe asthma, it is very important that he obtains the help of a well-trained allergist or chest physician in his area. Asthmatics must learn to contact their physicians as early as possible when severe attacks begin so that serious distress can be prevented. The sooner an asthmatic attack is brought under control, the easier it is to treat. If a patient wheezes for many hours or days before the physician is contacted, it is much more difficult to stop the attack. Asthma is often especially severe at night. If an attack is severe and not improving, notify the doctor before he goes to bed rather than waiting till 2 or 3 A.M. Asthmatics who are vacationing or on holiday are definitely more at risk than at other times. (See page 233) for advice to help prevent serious problems when you are away from home.)

What should you do when you can't contact your physician?
Contact another physician or immediately go to the emergency department of the nearest large hospital.

INFECTION AND ASTHMA

What is an infection?
An infection is an illness caused by germs, usually either bacteria or viruses. The most frequent infection is a common cold or upper respiratory infection. Others affect the tonsils or throat, ears, chest or intestines. The initial asthma episode, as well as subsequent ones, may often be associated with an infection. It is not always easy to diagnose an infection. A patient may have pain, fever, or green or yellow mucus. Children and adults often have an infection and do not realize it. Usually a physician can detect infection but this is not always possible, especially when the infection first begins. Most children have 4 infections a year but allergic children may have an infection every 2 or 3 weeks, each one lasting about 10 days so that one barely subsides before the next starts.

What is a normal temperature?
By mouth the temperature should be approximately 37.0°C. By rectum the temperature should be 37.5°C. There is a normal daily variation, however, of approximately 0.5°C. Some people normally have a low temperature and this is seldom a point of concern. A rise of 0.5°C. is also not serious. If, however, the temperature rises above normal (more than 1°C.), this probably would indicate infection, not allergy. Most uncomplicated allergies would not cause a fever. A drug reaction or certain delayed allergic reactions could be exceptions. A patient can have an infection, such as viral pneumonia, and not have a fever.

Does an X-ray always reveal a lung infection?
Usually an X-ray would show pneumonia but not always. Early in the course of an infection when a physician might hear pneumonia, the X-ray might not reveal it. A few days later the X-ray might reveal pneumonia but the physician might be unable to detect it. Asthma patients do not need X-rays every time they wheeze, but certainly should have one when the wheeze is noticed for the first time. When a physician hears unusual sounds in any part of the lungs, he will order future chest X-rays.

Can asthma make you prone to infection?
In some patients it certainly can. Germs can be present normally in everyone's nose and throat. If the tissues swell because of allergies, germs

can invade more readily, possible because of an inadequate blood supply. When asthma is well-treated, tissues are less swollen and infections are less apt to occur.

In some individuals infections may precipitate asthma without really causing it. (See page 6). Normally a certain amount of exposure to allergenic substances is necessary before symptoms occur. If someone has an infection, less exposure to allergenic substances is necessary before asthmatic episodes are triggered.

Many patients may develop an infection and begin to wheeze within a few hours. If this pattern is typical, it means that at the first sign of an infection, asthma medicine should be given. This may help prevent wheezing. Many asthmatics wheeze with almost every infection. Efforts must be made to prevent this. The duration of asthma often can be shortened if both an antibiotic and drugs to control asthma are given. The sooner "both" drugs are started, the sooner the attack is under control. Remember, however, that viral infections are not helped by antibiotics.

After a patient has responded to comprehensive allergy treatment, he may be able to get an infection and not wheeze or need asthma drugs or an antibiotic.

How can family infections be decreased?

We cannot readily explain why some parents who take good care of their family have one infection after another, while other families whose care is far from exemplary, have well children. These are a few measures which *might* prove helpful in decreasing infections in some families:

1. Use Lysol or an antiseptic in cleaning water.

2. Be certain that infected persons cover their mouths when they cough and frequently wash their hands.

3. Be certain that dishes and silverware are rinsed with boiling water.

4. Be certain that each family member has his own drinking glass.

5. Have all family members gargle daily with an antiseptic mouth wash each morning and evening when any member of the family has a cold.

6. Allergic individuals often become very ill with each infection. When another member of the family becomes ill, he should avoid contact with the allergic person if at all possible.

Do infections cause asthma?

Many physicians believe that some adults and children are allergic to bacteria or germs or products these organisms form in the body. This type of allergy is difficult to treat. It is sometimes called "intrinsic" asthma. (See page 33). One way to treat intrinsic asthma associated with infection is to give antibiotics. Another way is to give respiratory or bacterial vaccines but strong controversy exists regarding this form of therapy. Some physicians have not found bacterial vaccines helpful.

EMOTIONS IN ASTHMA

Do parents overprotect an asthmatic child?

If every time a child goes outside to play in the cold or becomes fatigued or tired he begins to wheeze, it does not take long before a parent realizes this youngster is different and starts to limit his activities. The child may be overdressed and not allowed to play normally. This is not really overprotection but common sense adjustment to a difficult situation. Most parents will allow their child to act like other youngsters as soon as he is able.

If, however, a parent limits a youngster's activities and overdresses him *after* the allergies are well-controlled, this is overprotection. The physician will help decide when a child can be treated normally.

Do parents contribute to their child's asthma?

Parents certainly do not knowingly make their child wheeze. Sometimes, however, parents are frightened when they see their child wheezing. If a parent trembles or is about to cry, this makes a youngster's asthma worse. A child can sense a parent's fear by small changes reflected in the face or tone of the voice. If you have ever been truly frightened, you know it is extremely difficult to breathe. A wheezing child already has difficulty breathing, so fright added to the asthma worsens the situation. Try to be calm and give your youngster the correct medicine. If this does not help, contact your physician or take your child to the nearest hospital.

Do special problems arise with divorced or separated parents?

This situation often causes difficulties in allergic children. The asthmatic youngster may be fine until he visits the separated parent. Because of multiple factors such as a different environment, exposure to an animal, anxiety, and dietary lapses, the child returns home sick with asthma. This may happen repeatedly and is difficult to prevent. The child may be unconsciously used as a means of "getting back at the mate".

The best treatment is to give asthma drugs before visits. The physician has the obligation to educate both parents as much as possible concerning all aspects of the child's illness. At times it is possible for a father to be a better parent for his allergic child than a loving but extremely nervous mother.

Do emotions cause asthma:
There is much controversy about this among physicians. Many feel that an infection, similar to an emotional upset, irritating fumes, or exertion merely *trigger* asthmatic episodes, (See pages 43 to 52) but that none of these really *cause* wheezing. Once a child has responded well to allergy management, these previous triggering factors cause less difficulty and asthma will not routinely be associated with each exposure.
It is hard to find a family where recurrent emotional problems or stresses aren't present. One must be cautious not to attribute every illness that cannot readily be explained to emotional factors within a family. There is no doubt, however, that in some children and adults, emotions can be a factor, and in a few nervous factors seem to be a major triggering mechanism. (See page 6).

Does asthma cause emotional problems?
A severely asthmatic individual is definitely limited and restricted in many ways. Is it the asthma, however, which causes emotional problems or the reverse? It is possible that some psychological problems resolve themselves once the patient has responded to allergy treatment. Some individuals, however, respond poorly and might need psychiatric help in accepting the fact that they do have a chronic illness. An asthmatic, like a person who has diabetes, arthritis or any serious chronic disabling illnessess may justifiably need help in accepting the fact that they are different.

How can wheezing upset children be relaxed?
Youngsters often wheeze, become upset and cry. The more upset they become, the more severe the asthma is.
It becomes a vicious cycle. Sedatives or sleep producing medicines cause drowsiness but should be avoided because they could interfere with breathing. (See page 108). It might lessen anxiety if a child were given 2 or 3 teaspoons of wine or whisky in a sweetened fruit juice. This should not be used often or in excess. The youngster should *not be told* what "medicine" he is being given. This helps quiet a child and the wheezing is reduced without interference with the child's breathing.

Can some children wheeze whenever they desire?
Some children (and adults) can. Young children will verbalize openly that if they aren't given something immediately they will wheeze and promptly proceed to carry out their threat. The solution of this problem is not easy. Immediately give an asthma medicine and in 20 minutes, or sooner if necessary, treat this child like a youngster who did not have asthma.

The vicious cycle must be broken. Try not to give in to the demands of the child. If much is to be gained by wheezing, and a child can wheeze at will, a most undesirable personality pattern may ensue. At times short or long stay institutional treatment may be necessary to break this type of behaviour.

When giving reprimands, it is superior to deny something in the form of play or sweets than to use physical punishment. Parents must not make idle threats which they do not or cannot enforce or the child will continually be challenging their authority. The child must learn that his illness cannot be used for personal gains. If a child threatens to wheeze because his parents are going out for an evening, the parents must be firm. The sitter must know exactly how to treat an asthma attack and parents should check frequently to be certain that all is well. The child must realize that parents too have rights. Once a youngster has responded well to allergy treatment, emotions are much less likely to trigger attacks.

MISCELLANEOUS FACTORS RELATED TO ASTHMA

Do breathing exercises help asthma?

Breathing exercises help patients control their wheezing and to breathe more effectively. This type of exercise is for the severe chronic asthmatic. A booklet called "Exercises for Asthma and Emphysema" (See page 261) is written for both adults and children. It helps if a hospital physiotherapist, trained to teach adults or children, initially shows them how to do the exercises and breathing manoeuvres. The patient must learn to breathe using the lower rib cage or chest. He must try to breathe out more air than he breathes in. Children can play games such as blowing up balloons or blowing a ping pong ball across a table at some target. This helps to reduce excess air trapped in the lungs during asthmatic episodes. The best and most natural way to learn correct breathing is to swim properly and regularly in adequately warm water.

Can an asthmatic play wind musical instruments?

An asthmatic who learns to play a wind instrument correctly will be doing breathing exercises. Smaller instruments are best. Some years ago, this type of activity was felt to be harmful but this is no longer true.

Will asthma cause deformities of the chest?

Wheezing children seldom have chest deformities. Severe wheezes, however, cause excessive air trapping in the lungs and the chest becomes more rounded. When the attack stops, the excess air leaves the lungs and the chest contour becomes more normal. Some asthmatics have a caved in or "funnel" chest or a prominent projected chest – "pigeon chest". The lower chest may be pulled in and appear flattened from constant muscular effort to breathe in. Those who have had extreme severe wheezing for long periods of time, such as 10 or 15 years, will have this "pulled in" appearance. Adults who have wheezed for many years can have permanently rounded shoulders and a so called "barrel" chest due to air trapping. Some asthmatics become permanently wheezy with continued cough and spasm which cannot be relieved. These patients have developed chronic bronchitis in addition to their asthmatic condition. Usually they are cigarette smokers.

How important is tobacco smoke in relation to asthma?

Tobacco smoke can trigger asthma, regardless of who is doing the smoking. It can act both as a chemical and mechanical irritation. The sooner a person with lung problems gives up smoking, the greater the chances for improving the breathing. Tobacco pollution will definitely increase the tendency to develop infection such as bronchitis or emphysema which are difficult to treat. Exposure to tobacco smoke of any type will damage lungs. Persons who wheeze for any reason, *MUST not smoke.*

Does asthma affect the heart?

Children can wheeze for prolonged periods of time without measurable objective evidence to show any alteration in the heart or the lungs. Asthma can cause a faster heart beat but this is not any more harmful than having the child run down the street. X-rays show no specific abnormality found only in asthmatics. Only the exceptional asthmatic child shows significant changes on an electrocardiogram.

Adult asthmatics think that because they become breathless and blue with exertion and their pulse rate increases, that their heart must be affected. It is their lungs and not their heart that is the cause of their difficulty. An electrocardiogram will confirm the doctor's evaluation and should be routine for any adult asthmatic during his first hospital admission. Often, patients confuse this with cardiac asthma. This disease is due to high blood pressure affecting the heart which is causing difficult breathing. (See page 58). Some patients have bronchial asthma, others cardiac asthma.

Some asthma drugs, such as adrenaline, can increase the heart rate. These drugs, however, are now being replaced by superior medications which have little or no effect upon the heart rate.

How helpful is therapy given in spas?

Any special centre for treating asthma, teaches the patient a way of living with asthma. Special centres may stress a fine location such as at the seaside or in the mountains, but most spas have a treatment based on benefits received from special waters. The water is taken as a drink, sprayed on the skin and given as a mist to relieve congestion of the nose or chest. In Great Britain, there are no spas for the treatment of asthma, but in France many children go to La Bouboule and adults to LeMont d'Or for "the cure". In Germany, children may go to special spas.

How helpful is negative ionization treatment?

This method of treatment has been used in Russia for a number of years. There seems to be no acceptable scientific evidence that this method helps asthma.

Is hospitalization a problem for asthmatics?

If an asthma patient is hospitalized for any reason, his room should be as allergy-free as possible. If available, an air-purifier (See page 151) can be placed in the bedroom. The mattress and box springs should be entirely encased in plastic and the pillow must be synthetic. Woollen blankets should not be used.

It is difficult to follow a diet in a hospital because many persons care for one sick individual. Even though everyone is supposed to know that a patient cannot drink milk or eat eggs, always recheck the tray before eating. Significant errors are often made.

Can surgery be a problem for an asthmatic?

In general, if patients are not wheezing when they enter the hospital and if they stay in an allergy-free room and use their asthma drugs when needed, surgery presents no special problems. The indications for removal of an appendix, tonsils, adenoids or teeth are basically the same in allergic or non-allergic persons. The following, however, should be remembered:

1. Tonsils and adenoids should not be removed during a pollen season from anyone who has nose allergies but has never wheezed. Asthma is sometimes started for the first time after an operation during a pollen season. (See page 83).

2. If a patient has been using cortisone or steroids (See page 110) this should be discussed with your physician, surgeon and anaesthetist. Additional steroids might be necessary prior to surgery to combat the stress of an operation. (See page 111). The decision concerning this would depend upon the amount and times when a patient received cortisone.

3. All efforts must be made to continue a patient's usual diet while he is in the hospital.

4. Another consideration is that surgery makes anyone anxious and upset. It is helpful prophylactically to use a long acting asthma drug the night before surgery unless this is contraindicated, to help prevent morning asthma. If wheezing were noted, adrenaline could be given. No

drugs should be taken on the day of surgery unless your physician specified to do so.

5 It is possible to have an allergic reaction to an anaesthetic or to certain types of X-rays using iodides. There is no way to accurately test in advance to tell whether the patient is allergic to them or not. If a drug is known to be safe, this should be used in preference to one which possibly caused trouble in the past. Adults who have nose polyps and a sensitivity to aspirin seem particularly liable to develop more drug allergies, e.g. penicillin. Be sure to tell the physician in charge, the surgeon and the anaesthetist about any episodes of possible drug reactions. Errors about drug allergies can cause alarming or fatal results.

Providing caution is taken to inform both the medical and surgical doctors about a patient's allergic problems, and wheezing is not present at the time of surgery, most tolerate surgery well.

Should asthmatic children engage in sports?

Asthmatic children can engage in any sports activity providing they are not obviously having difficulty breathing. They may, however, need to take asthma medicine before they start to exercise, if activity usually causes wheezing. If a child wheezes badly in spite of having taken his medicine prior to play, exercise would have to be limited until the allergies were better controlled.

If limitation of activity is necessary it helps if children learn judo, weight lifting, karate, or some activity which not only improves their body and self image but makes them feel superior.

Asthmatic children do very well when they swim. An Olympic gold medallist had asthma. Swimming may not be the only sport which will not cause an asthmatic to wheeze. Any form of play, however, which entails short bursts of activity, such as basketball or football, may be well tolerated. Asthmatics do well if they play hard for a few minutes and then rest. They do poorly, however, in physical fitness tests which require repetitive activity until exhaustion. Asthmatic children should be cautioned not to try to excel in this type of activity.

Asthmatic youngsters of normal size should not diet or use diuretics so they fall into certain weight categories for wrestling or ball sports. Their body weight should be maintained at what is best for their health and not at some level required for some sport's activity.

Should adult asthmatics exercise?

Adult asthmatics may know from experience that strenuous exercise makes them wheeze. They may mistakenly give up all forms of sports and exercise. The only restriction an adult asthmatic should have would be dictated by what nature allows. If exercise has to be limited, the diet should also be limited. An asthmatic adult should be thin rather than fat.

Which occupations should an asthmatic select?
  Asthmatics should earn their livelihood by entering careers which
would not make allergies worse. They definitely should not become
beauticians or barbers, firemen, painters, bakers, garage mechanics,
taxidermists, policemen, veterinarians, or farmers. They must avoid
occupations which expose them to cold weather, excessive moisture or
dampness, heavy air pollution, excessive dust or irritating odours. Any
occupation requiring hard physical work is not advisable. A farmer will
not do any farm chore which he knows will cause asthma. If he is in
charge there is no problem; it is when he is not in charge, that difficulty
arises. In general, an office job of some sort suits asthmatics. The nearer
the job is to his home, the less travelling there will be. Long distance travelling to work on very hot or cold days can be difficult for asthmatics.

How can you make a severe asthmatic feel superior?
  To feel superior, you need to be superior in some way. Special study or
training in anything will make you better. Any mental, artistic, or physical endeavour which makes you better than most people, would be
helpful. Musical or creative talent should be encouraged. For mental
stimulation, chess or bridge might give additional self esteem and satisfaction.
  If sports are preferred, engage in any of the activities previously mentioned. Sometimes photography, knitting, designing or sewing are
helpful.

Will a move to another part of your country help asthma?
  The response to any move will depend upon what is causing the
asthma. If it is a food which will be eaten anywhere, the problem will
remain. If the cause is something that will be carried with the family,
such as a pillow, mattress, pet, or favourite overstuffed chair, the problems may continue in the new home.
  If a person is pollen sensitive, it is difficult to find an area which will
not have pollen. All pollen is not similar but pollen sensitive patients can
develop an allergy to excessive or prolonged new pollen exposure.
  To move a family to a distant area, leaving relatives and friends, and
finding new employment, are such drastic measures that all possible
factors must be throughly considered. A move might be of value if a
person lived in an unusually heavily pollinated area, if this pollen were
his special problem. If the problem is your home, it is better to simply
move to a new house within your present area.
  Some patients who move to distant areas with different climates
sometimes do surprisingly well. One cannot predict the response,
however, of any particular patient.
  Coastal asthma in Africa is often due to household dust mites which

are found in the moist warm coast and not found in the drier high parts, e.g. Johannesburgh. Remember asthma is a world-wide problem.

Will asthma affect a child's growth?

Asthmatic youngsters, unless they are constantly ill, grow as well as other children. If a child needs daily rather than every other day steroids, (See page 112) for prolonged periods of time, growth can definitely be less than normal. If steroids or cortisone are discontinued before puberty, there is a compensatory growth spurt and normal height will be attained. Cortisone in itself can cause weight gain and make the face look very round, but this is usually a temporary change. (See page 112).

Should allergic couples limit the size of their families?

Genetic counselling of medical advice concerning raising a family is given for very few inherited diseases. The hereditary aspects of allergic disease are barely beginning to be understood. If both parents are highly "allergic", one would anticipate an increase of allergic diseases in their children.

Sometimes, two or more members of a family may have to receive allergy treatment, but rarely would more than one member be a severe and difficult allergic patient to treat. Identical twins may not both have allergies.

If you have allergies and take precautions when you start housekeeping, it may be possible to delay or prevent this problem in your youngster. If, however, you furnish your home with feathers, wool and pets, you can rest less easily in this regard. (See page 137).

What is baker's asthma?

There is one type of wheezing which commonly occurs in bakers and is caused by exposure to wheat flour in particular, but also from rye or corn flour. These patients do not have symptoms from eating baked goods which contain flour.

What is hypersensitivity pneumonitis?

This type of wheezing is noted mainly in adults. It is caused by any fine dust such as from moulds found in association with hay, sugar cane, maple bark, cheese, malt, cork or dust from furnaces, air conditioners, and humidifiers. Both the spores and dust from a mushroom compost can cause symptoms from the dust and excreta. Fine sawdust, particularly from redwood, also causes this problem.

Characteristically, 4 to 6 hours after exposure, the sensitive person develops fever and chills, aches, pains, cough and shortness of breath. Attacks may last from hours to days or weeks. Some patients have weight loss and a poor appetite. Between episodes patients may seem quite well.

They may incorrectly believe they have had bronchitis due to infection. Symptoms may disappear each week-end or on holidays if the problem is entirely related to dust exposure at work. Pigeon fanciers, whose contact could be mainly on weekends, would be worse mainly at that time. Delayed allergy skin tests are sometimes helpful in the diagnosis. Filtering masks or proper ventilation of contaminated areas may help temporarily but if the patient is extremely ill, *complete* avoidance of exposure and steroids (cortisone) may be necessary.

What is aspergillosis?

This is a complication of allergic asthma caused by a mould. The patients often have X-ray changes which come and go and look like pneumonia. The sputum is yellow or green and may become blood stained. These patients have a special type of bronchiectasis (See page 58). It is diagnosed by sputum study, skin tests and X-ray. They are sometimes treated with cortisone drugs but antibiotics are seldom helpful.

What are some non-allergic causes of wheezing?

There are so many causes that a physician is needed to determine why anyone wheezes. Wheezing at any age can be caused by anything which is in the lungs preventing the easy passage of air through the airtubes or by anything which presses against the outside of the air passageways (causing an indentation into the breathing tubes). Common causes are as follows:

1. FOREIGN ITEMS IN THE LUNG

In the first two years of life in particular wheezing can be caused by many problems unrelated to allergies. It is very important to be sure that a foreign object such as a button or bone did not accidentally get into a young child's lungs. This can also happen to older children or adults during choking episodes when eating. Remember that all swallowed objects will not be seen on an X-ray. Metal, plastic or bone will usually be seen, but foods such as peanuts or organic substances such as weeds would not be seen.

2. INFECTION

One of the most common causes of non-allergic wheezing is lung infection which sometimes eventually can cause chronic bronchitis. Such patients often have a history of coughing for years and their sputum is discoloured (either yellow, green or grey) and possibly blood-tinged. Between wheezing episodes these patients often have breathlessness and

just prior to the start of a wheezing episode, a new infection may be noted. Infection causing bronchitis often occurs without a fever.
Infection within the lungs can eventually lead to bronchiectasis and emphysema (See page 59). Bronchiectasis is a chronic infection of the smaller outermost divisions of the lungs called bronchioles or smaller bronchi. These tiny air tubes lose their shape, become stretched, and are often filled with puddles of infection which can extend into the walls of the lung tubes. Patients who have bronchiectasis cough up green and yellow mucus and occasionally blood. They often have a foul odour to their breath and to the mucus which they spit up. They sometimes also have a chronic sinus infection. X-ray of the inside of the lungs (bronchography) (See page 212) confirms the diagnosis of bronchiectasis. Lung physiotherapy which includes postural drainage is a necessary part of patient care (See page 51). Prompt prolonged treatment of infection with an antibiotic is essential for proper treatment. Surgical removal of badly affected portions of the lungs is also occasionally needed.

Asthmatic bronchitis means different things to different people and doctors. Usually, however, it means that a patient has a combination of intermittent asthma or wheezing associated with some element of infection.

3. NON-SPECIFIC BRONCHITIS

This type of wheezing is due mainly to exposure to irritating substances such as certain dusts, tobacco smoke and air pollution, such as volatile chemicals and very cold air.

4. CANCER OR TUMORS

Tumor growths, in or near the lungs, due to cancer or benign (non cancerous) growths, can prevent the normal flow of air to and from the lungs and cause wheezing. X-rays or bronchoscopy (looking inside the air tubes. (See page 212) are helpful in diagnosing such problems.

5. HEART DISEASE

Some patients with heart disease develop cardiac asthma. This condition can mimic allergic asthma very closely. It usually starts in middle age. It is caused in part by a strain on the heart. The heart pump circulates blood. As blood is returned from distant portions of the body to the lungs, carbon dioxide is removed and oxygen is added. In these patients the heart pump can't move the blood efficiently through the lungs. Some of these patients definitely have a mixture of allergic asthma, heart disease and infection. In those patients who have an allergic component, removal of allergenic offending substances can be helpful.

The symptoms of cardiac asthma occur most often at night during sleep. The patient complains of a feeling of suffocation and has great difficulty breathing in *and* out (asthmatics usually have much more difficulty breathing out, than in). Cardiac asthma may cause an ashen face colour. Patients may perspire although they are not warm. Attacks last about one hour but can vary from a few minutes to several hours. Afterwards the patients are exhausted, at times for many hours. There are many ways to treat this type of asthma. Follow your doctor's recommendations.

Can asthma cause emphysema?

Children who have chronic severe asthma can have marked air-trapping and possibly a reversible pre-emphysema.

Adults who have chronic asthma complicated by infection can develop emphysema. Emphysema means the small balloon sponge-like sections of the lungs loose their elasticity. The sectors that divide the little portions of the lungs become broken down by infection. Some sections may balloon out and become too large and the compartments separating the little divisions may break down. Mucus cannot be eliminated properly and infection becomes a problem. Because the lung sectors are not as elastic as normal, air cannot be forced out as effectively. This causes trapping of air in some sectors and a lack of air in others.

In general, emphysema patients will have shortness of breath when they are not wheezing and will tend to have more difficulty breathing especially when they exert themselves or if they are exposed to cold, wind, or dust. Affected persons often speak in short choppy phrases because of their difficulty trying to breathe while talking. Chronic emphysema can follow or precede chronic bronchitis. Prolonged infection in asthmatics is only one cause of emphysema.

It is often difficult to tell the difference between allergic asthma and bronchitis, with or without emphysema, because all of these conditions can coexist simultaneously. Smoking makes all these lung problems worse.

CHAPTER FOUR

Eczema

What is eczema?
Eczema is a general term referring to many skin rashes. In this chapter the term eczema means atopic dermatitis. It refers only to a special type of itchy skin rash frequently seen in allergic infants, children and sometime in adults. Most eczema is worse during the colder months, but about 20 per cent of patients are worse during the warm weather. It is not contagious.

Eczema is not present at birth, but infants often have the first signs of the rash on the cheeks or body by 3 or 6 months of age. As a child becomes older, the rash often localizes to the arm or leg creases or the wrists, lower arms, calves and ankles. It sometimes affects the entire body, but the buttocks and upper inner arms are often spared. The rash can cause coin-shaped (nummular) body spots. In older children, the skin in the arm and leg creases and the back of the neck tends to become thicker and darker than normal. The finger tips are also scaly and cracked.

Without any specific treatment, eczema may clear by the age of 2 or 3 years. Children who have had this problem often have dry skin throughout their lives. The upper outer arms may be rough and slightly bumpy. At or before puberty, eczema can change becoming better in some patients and worse in others. In about 25 per cent of severely affected children, eczema persists well into adult life.

If an infant's skin is very soft, there is a better chance that eczema will not be severe or prolonged. If eczema starts very early in infancy and is very severe, it is more apt to be a lifetime problem. There are many exceptions, however.

What causes eczema?
No one knows for sure, but it is *believed* that eczema may be due to the same factors which cause other allergies. Inhaled substances such as dust (mites), animal hair (dandruff, wool, feathers), mould spores, pollens

and perfumed substances are believed to be factors in some individuals. Foods seem to be of particular significance in infants although many physicians do not agree that foods are related to this problem. Pollens are seldom a factor until after the age of 2 years.

Is there any way to prevent eczema?

Because we do not know exactly what causes it, it is not easy to prevent the rash. Avoid any substances which obviously or possibly make it worse. Some studies indicate that breast feeding is less apt to be followed by eczema in very allergic families than the use of cow's milk. General measures which help to decrease eczema are listed on page 110. The elimination of highly allergenic substances from your home is explained in Chapter 11 and Chapter 12 contains specific advice concerning how to check for food allergy.

How can the cause of an eczema outbreak be determined?

Watch the child who has eczema, especially when he is eating or playing. If scratching suddenly begins in the arm or leg creases, or in any skin area, it could indicate a recent exposure to something causing the rash. The skin, however, might not show eczema until the next day. A parent can check any suspicious factor by purposely exposing the youngster to that item in the future, and noticing if exposure repeatedly flares the skin problem.

An individual's skin can be almost perfect and suddenly the eczema reappears. Each day the skin becomes progressively worse. The answer to the problem lies in remembering details about *the day before* the rash was first evident. Was there any unusual or different exposure? Were strange contacts made on that day, or was anything unusual eaten? It helps to make a list of everything you can recall which might possibly be a factor related to the flare. Any factors such as unusual emotional upsets, exertion, or overheating might in someway be related to the new eczema rash.

An allergist will try to relate any major flare-up of the skin to exposure to possible allergenic substances. A careful history is essential in helping your physician solve this difficult skin problem. Parents of eczema children or adults who have this problem can eventually become very keen and perceptive if they begin to think about what might have caused a recurrence of the rash.

At what age does eczema begin?

Although eczema most frequently starts early in infancy, it can begin at any age. It sometimes appears quite suddenly but unfortunately seldom disappears quickly.

What sex has more eczema?
More boys than girls have eczema during infancy and early childhood, while girls predominate in later childhood and in adults.

Do other allergies develop in persons who have eczema?
A child who develops eczema has a 50 per cent chance of developing some other forms of allergies by the age of 10 years. Usually these affect the nose (hay fever) or chest (asthma). It may be possible to delay or prevent the development of future allergies *if* allergy precautions are carried out as suggested in Chapter 11.

Which eczema infants are apt to develop more allergies?
Subsequent allergies are more likely to develop if:
1.   There are many relatives in that baby's family who have allergies.
2.   The eczema in the affected baby is very severe.
3.   The eczema began very early in infancy.
4.   The infant with eczema cannot eat eggs.
5.   The infant has evidence within his blood of having strong allergies.
(See page 121).

How should salves be applied to the skin of a person with eczema?
A salve can be applied locally to the skin as often as prescribed by your physician. Proper application implies the use of tiny amounts several times a day.
A small amount of salve should be placed on the tip of the finger. Apply tiny specks every ½ inch over the affected skin, then rub the specks together. This type of application covers the skin with an even, thin coating more effectively and inexpensively than a thick application once a day. Expensive eczema salves should not be applied like cold cream. Most should be applied at least four times a day. Many contain steroids.

Are steroids (cortisones) safe when applied on the skin?
When steroids are part of a skin salve, they seldom cause undesirable effects. When very large areas of a baby, however, are affected with wet oozing eczema, some types of steroids can be absorbed and cause side effects (See page 112). More cortisone is absorbed when it is applied and covered with a special type of clear thin colourless plastic. This sometimes is used to help heal the skin more quickly. Long continued use of certain strong cortisone creams applied to the face is sometimes not advisable.
Cortisone taken by mouth or by injection can be dangerous under certain circumstances (See page 112). Used in this manner, it will often eliminate eczema but when the dose is decreased, the eczema may become very bad, possibly worse than it was originally. For this reason

cortisone is seldom given by mouth or by injection, except when the physician feels that the eczema is an unusually difficult problem to treat. (See page 111).

Can a skin salve make eczema worse?

It is possible for a person's skin to itch or burn immediately after applying an ointment. If this happens, the treatment should be stopped until you discuss this with your physician. The burning may be eliminated by wetting the skin slightly with water before applying the cream, but the burning or itch often indicates some ingredient in the ointment is bothering the skin. If the skin appears to be worse the day following use of a new skin treatment, it should not be continued until you have checked with your physician.

It is a wise precaution when using a new skin preparation to apply it to an obscure 2 inch area of skin. Wait at least a half a day before applying it to large areas of the body to be sure there is no sensitivity to some component in the salve.

Do antihistamines, taken by mouth, help eczema?

They help but we often can't explain why. They may only make a patient sleepy, or may decrease the itchiness of the skin. Many patients scratch mainly at night. It helps if a long acting 8 to 12 hour antihistamine is taken at bedtime. Many antihistamines cause children and adults to become sleepy and these are excellent to use just before retiring. (See page 104).

Can a child, who has eczema all over the body, be skin tested?

Yes. The upper inner arm is usually clear and that small area can be used for allergy skin testing if necessary.

Are allergy skin tests helpful?

Food skin tests are not always of value because they may not be reliable. It is possible to have a positive food skin reaction and not have any symptoms when the food is eaten or a negative skin reaction when allergy exists. Other tests, especially for pollens or moulds which can cause eczema to worsen during the warm months, would be helpful.

Does allergy extract treatment help eczema?

Allergy-injection therapy may help the type of eczema which is worse during the warmer months, when tree, grass and weed pollens are evident, and when mould spores are a problem. The more typical patient who has a flare of his eczema during the cold months is often not helped. *Occasionally*, however, patients being treated for year-round asthma and hay fever, find that their eczema clears dramatically.

It is possible for allergy-extract therapy to cause eczema to become

worse. Sometimes a day or two after an injection treatment, the skin
worsens. If this happens the treatments often can be continued if the
allergy extract medicine is made weaker or less is given during each
treatment. Your physician can advise you in this regard.

How can the itch associated with eczema be decreased?

1. Medicines called antihistamines (See page 103) tend to decrease
itching. On occasion, however, several antihistamines may have to be
tried before one is found which helps. (See page 103). These medicines are
available in both liquid and pill forms and are taken by mouth. Antihistamines should *not* be applied directly to the skin because this can
cause an allergy to develop to the antihistamine in that preparation.

2. The itch is decreased if the skin is treated with a preparation which
contains a tar. This ingredient changes the colour of a white cream to a
tan or brownish colour.

Is eczema made worse from contact with water?

There is some difference of opinion about this among allergists and
dermatologists, but in general water does not seem to make the skin
worse. For example, many children can swim for long periods every day
during the warm months and their skin is not worse. When swimming in
pools, they are exposed not only to water but to the many chemicals in it.
It is believed that soap, or possibly scouring powder left in the tub after
cleaning could irritate the skin.

Can a patient's eczema become worse during infection?

Colds and certain viral infections can make eczema worse. Measles,
however, is often associated with an improvement in eczema. Patients
who develop cold sores when they have eczema can sometimes become
quite ill. (See page 68).

Is there any special soap which is best for someone who has eczema?

A mild soap which is not alkaline is best. Although most commercial
soaps are alkaline, some are mild and your physician can recommend
which are best. More expensive non-allergic soaps can be obtained from
chemists. Perfumed soaps should not be used because these can cause
allergies. Some soaps contain lanolin which sometimes causes eczema to
become worse.

Will eczema improve if you don't bathe?

There are some dermatologists who recommend this. The skin is
cleansed with certain lotions or soap substitutes. Water is not put on the
skin for a prolonged period of time, and eventually the skin may become
softer and more oily.

Is there any laundry soap which would be best for patients with eczema?
A laundry soap which contains strong brightening and bleaching agents would be inferior to a mild soap. Use the mild laundry soap suggested by your physician for all clothing, including towels, sheets and pillow cases.

Housewives should check the rinse cycle after washing clothing to see if the last rinse water is entirely clear. It is not uncommon to find that last rinse to be cloudy indicating that the clothing should be re-rinsed or the entire wash and rinse cycle repeated without using any soap.

Are there any special recommendations about bathing and eczema?
Soap tends to irritate eczema skin so little should be used. The entire skin cannot be sudsed thoroughly every day. This would dry the skin, and cause more scratching and eczema. During the colder months of the year patients bathe ever week or two but during the warmer months, bathing can be more frequent. Some physicians believe it is not harmful to bathe in water without soap. A tepid shower definitely would be preferable to long soaks in soapy water.

A child with eczema should never take a bubble bath or place detergent in the bath water because these could dry the skin. Young children tend to use an excessive amount of bubble producing items.

Extremely hot water should be avoided. Anything which causes overheating could increase the tendency to itch and scratch.

Oatmeal and starch are sometimes added to baths to make the skin feel better. One or two cups of cornstarch and one cup of soda (sodium bicarbonate) per tub of bath water is sometimes beneficial. An emulsifying ointment can be made into a thin cream and poured into the bath water. The ointment can also be used on the skin instead of soap. Check with your physician.

Do bath oils help dry skin?
If an oil is placed in a tub of warm water, the oil accumulates along the edges of the tub and makes the tub slippery and dangerous. If any oil happens to be on the skin it is wiped onto a soft bath towel. Little, therefore, stays on the skin if the oil is placed in the bath water. It is more effective to bathe and partially dry yourself before applying the oil unless contrary suggestions are made by your physician.

What general measures help eczema?
A. Patients with eczema should avoid overheating because increased perspiration causes itching and scratching. Extreme exertion, anxiety, or emotional upsets, or an overheated home or bedroom can make eczema

worse. Avoid locating the bed near the bedroom's source of heat. Hot baths cause overheating.

B. The fingernails should be kept very short and clean to decrease the tendency to damage the skin and introduce infection. The nails should be filed as short as possible twice a week so that no white shows on the outer edge of the nail. Any sharp points or jagged edges must be filed. At night, it is sometimes helpful if a child wears mittens or socks over his hands, or even boxing gloves. No attempt should be made to tie down a child's arms and legs when he is in bed to prevent itching. Older children and adults know that they should not scratch but this cannot be avoided because their skin is often extremely itchy.

C. Persons with eczema should wear smooth clothing, preferably loose weave cottons. They should avoid rough fabrics, wool, or synthetic preparations which increase perspiration. Parents should avoid wearing wool when they hold and cuddle their youngster. Loose-fitting clothing is superior to tight-fitting clothing, which would not allow for free circulation of air about the skin. Zippered sleeping garments and warm flannel pyjamas should be avoided. Fabrics which contain animal hair should not be worn. Coloured clothing is better than white which would need bleaching. Children with foot eczema should not walk barefoot or wear only socks when they are inside their home.

D. Try to increase the humidity to normal within your home because skin affected by eczema tends to lose more moisture than normal and this is one reason why it is too dry.

E. It has been found that changes in environment often help patients who have eczema. For example, if a patient is hospitalized, the skin often clears. If a patient goes on a vacation to a warm dry climate, the skin will usually clear. The problem, however, is that upon return to the original home, the skin problem recurs again. (See page 8). To eliminate the skin problems at home, make your home more allergy-free.

F. Exposure to sunlight in moderation is believed to be beneficial for patients who have eczema. They must, however, be careful not to become overheated, to perspire excessively, or to become sunburned.

What special problems arise with eczema?

Infection is a frequent and sometimes serious problem. Scratching with dirty fingernails is one cause. The lymph nodes or glands in the armpits or the groin (where the upper leg meets the abdomen) become swollen and tender. Depending upon the severity of the infection, your physician might prescribe either a skin antibiotic or an antibiotic to be taken by mouth to help eliminate the infection. Anyone who has tender swollen lymph nodes or glands should be examined by their doctor. It is possible to be very ill and not to have a fever.

Does chronic eczema cause any unusual problems?
Persons who have had severe eczema for a period of over 10 years
rarely develop cataracts. An eye physician (that is an ophthalmologist,
not an optician or optometrist) could best advise an individual who had
this problem and remove the cataracts surgically if that were required.

Should someone who has eczema be vaccinated for smallpox?
No person who has eczema and no member of that person's family
should be vaccinated for smallpox unless the skin of the eczema patient
is ENTIRELY clear of ANY skin problem. Persons who have eczema
must avoid all contact with someone who has recently been vaccinated
unless the scab has fallen off the vaccination site. Parents must be careful
not to place a child with eczema into bath water used for a recently vaccinated child.
If someone, who has eczema, must be vaccinated, there is a special
effective and safe method available. Check with your physician.

Can an unvaccinated person who has eczema travel abroad?
It would depend entirely upon the regulations in the country in which
you live. You would have to check with your local health department
regarding the requirements in your country.
Smallpox is a problem at the present time in parts of Afghanistan,
Brazil, Congo (Dem. Rep.), Ethiopia, India, Indonesia, Kenya, Nepal,
West Pakistan, Bangladesh, South Africa and Sudan.

What is the relationship between scratching and eczema?
Eczema is always extremely itchy and this makes the patient scratch.
The itchy sensation can be triggered by something as slight as a change in
temperature or a draught. If a broken arm is placed in a cast, the skin
protected by the cast will not develop eczema. This is noted even though
the patient is exposed to something which causes eczema on other body
parts. Scratching, therefore, not only causes but aggravates eczema.

What is the difference between a cream and an ointment?
A cream is whitish in colour and similar to cold cream. An ointment
is very greasy, cloudy and is grey in colour. In general, ointments tend to
be less well tolerated by eczema patients than creams. When a patient
receives treatment to apply directly upon the skin, it is usually mixed
with either a cream or an ointment, so that it can be spread upon the skin.
If a patient notices that either a cream or ointment seems to be better
tolerated by his skin, he should tell his physician.

Should a dermatologist or allergist care for eczema?
Many patients who have eczema need the help of both types of spe-

cialists. A dermatologist is a medical specialist who cares for the skin. The allergist may confine his practice mainly to the care of allergies affecting the lungs, nose, eyes, intestines and skin. While both types of physicians could offer advice concerning antihistamines and possibly diets, the allergists would probably be more able to determine why the skin was breaking out and could also be helpful in trying to prevent or at least delay the onset of other forms of allergies. The dermatologist would be more knowledgeable about skin ointments or salves.

While most patients have eczema which is worse during the winter months, some have a warm weather flare. The latter could be due to pollens or mould spores and possibly would be helped by skin testing and hyposensitization.

Are there any precautions regarding other immunizations in relation to persons who have eczema?

In general, most patients who have eczema can tolerate the usual diphtheria, tetanus, or polio immunization procedures. The major precaution would be for an individual whose eczema worsens after contact with eggs. He should avoid receiving any vaccine which was grown on an egg media or base. This does *not* mean that a patient cannot receive a vaccine grown on eggs if he has a positive egg allergy skin test reaction. Vaccines grown on eggs would only have to be avoided by those individuals who *develop allergies when they eat or are near eggs*. Some recent research, however, would indicate that under certain circumstances even these individuals might be able to tolerate such vaccines. Your physician will advise you.

Measles vaccine may upset the eczema-asthma child. Until more is known about this vaccine, it might occasionally be necessary to withhold measles vaccine protection in such children. Check with your doctor.

Can a simple cold sore cause difficulty in a patient who has eczema?

It certainly can. The effect is very similar to that of exposure to a smallpox vaccination. The area of the skin affected by eczema and according to some reports, areas of the skin which have been affected by eczema in the past, can be worsened by the cold sore virus. Such patients are very ill and develop high temperatures. All persons who have eczema, regardless of their age, should be extremely careful to avoid not only contact with anyone who has recently had a smallpox vaccination but also contact with anyone who has a cold sore. This includes all members of the family, as well as friends. Although only a very small percentage of eczema patients exposed to cold sores develop complicating skin problems, caution in this regard must be stressed.

What is meant by contact dermatitis?

An allergic contact dermatitis may look similar to eczema however, when a contact dermatitis is first noted, tiny little blisters can be seen. Unlike typical eczema, a contact type dermatitis is usually not in the bends of the arms or legs. When a rash is due to contact, the affected skin is in the areas that are exposed to the contact. The face is often involved, as is the skin between the fingers or the tops of large toes.

Lipstick, cosmetics, perfumes and deodorants can all cause a rash in the area where they are applied to the skin. (See page 1). Nickel in watch straps, jewelry clips, and metallic fasteners used in ladies' undergarments can cause a rash in the area where the metal touches the skin. Rubber contact dermatitis is common and can be caused by rubber in shoes or in any garment which touches skin. Special adhesive bandage is sometimes necessary to cover small skin cuts if the usual adhesives cause a rash. Dyes used in clothing, or sprays and chemicals used in permanently pressed items, can cause dermatitis. The widow who dresses in black and develops a rash all over her body is suffering not from the effects of grief but from a contact dermatitis due to a black dye. Poison ivy, poison oak and sumac can cause a severe body rash when they come in contact with the skin of persons who have this type of sensitivity.

CHAPTER FIVE

Welts or nettle rash

What are welts or nettle rash?

This medical problem is called welts, nettle rash, hives or urticaria. These terms all refer to small red, itchy areas, on the skin. A raised, round whitish area in the centre may give the welt the appearance of a mosquito bite. A person can have a few welts or many scattered over his entire body. In order to develop an allergy (like welts) to a substance, previous exposure is necessary. Sometimes an allergy sensitivity quickly develops, at other times prolonged contact is needed. Sometimes adults have welts for many months, but most children and adults have only an occasional episode, for which there is no apparent cause.

There is one variant of welts which is called angioedema or angioneurotic edema (Quinke's oedema). This is a marked swelling of the deeper skin tissues, which does not itch but can hurt or cause a burning sensation. Although the skin may be red and swollen, the affected areas appear normal after the angioedema or welts are gone. This type of swelling can cause the face to become markedly distorted. The eyes may be mere slits and the lips, thick and large. Andioedema can cause so much swelling that the arms or legs may become rigid and hard to bend.

Regardless of what is causing the nettle rash or welts, they are made worse by overheating, hot baths or showers, exertion, emotional upsets, alcoholic drinks, and from pressure such as that due to a tight waist band or brassiere. Welts often occur in individuals who have no other obvious allergies.

Some people have skin which is sensitive when stroked. A blunt object rubbed along the skin will cause a raised, white line in the centre, and an area of redness on the edges. This does not indicate allergy, and is called dermographism. It is often a trait found in several members of certain families.

Is a single welt of significance?

Usually a single welt or a few welts are not really too important. Check the centre of the white raised area to see if there is a tiny hole in it. If the welt is due to an insect bite, there will be a definite opening in the centre.

How long do welts last?

A single episode of welts usually come and go for no apparent reason for several days or a week or two. If each day's reappearance of welts during a single episode seem less severe than the previous, and the flares come and go for only a couple of weeks, you should be relieved because this would indicate gradual improvement. Try not to be discouraged each time they reappear, providing this happens only for a couple of weeks. It is the exceptional patient who develops welts which persist for prolonged periods of time (six weeks to many years) and are a major challenge to treat. Most bouts of welts, especially in children, last only a few days and never recur. The cause is often not discovered, and because the episode occurs only once, it is no great cause of concern.

What most commonly causes welts or angioedema?

Sudden welts or angioedema which last a few days or weeks, are most often due to foods, drugs, various miscellaneous substances, and infection. Infrequent or unusual factors are commonly the cause of an isolated attack.

Chronic welts are those which are a problem for over 4 or 6 weeks. This type can recur or last for many years. Possible causes are drugs, infection, and foods. Frequent and continued exposure to some offending substance is most likely the cause of a prolonged problem.

Which foods commonly cause welts?

Frequently Cause Welts	
eggs	bananas
fish	peas
chocolate	pork
nuts (peanuts)	tomato products
shellfish	celery
fresh fruit (berries)	milk

Seldom Cause Welts		
alcohol ** (also in medicines)	gum	pickles
beans – of all types	licorice	preservatives for foods
carbonated beverages	mayonnaise	saccharin
cheese	meat sauces	seasonings
citrus fruits	menthol	spices

corn   mint   vegetables (fresh)
dyes – especially red or purple   mustard   wheat

**see pages 180, 185.

Which drugs are apt to cause welts?

Frequently Cause Welts

aspirin   hormones
penicillin   ACTH
barbiturates   insulin
codeine   oestrogens
                                  insulin
                                  pituitary extract
                                  thyroid preparations
                                  sulfonamides
                                  any type of antibiotic

Seldom Cause Welts

antihistamines   dyes (candy, canned   liver extract
atropine   fruits, gelatin,   mercurials
chloral hydrate   juices, margarine, morphine
coal tar derivative such as   medicines,   phenacetin
   acetanilide   vegetables, etc.) phenolphthalein
   antipyrine   eye, ear, and nose   derivatives
digitalis   drops   (laxatives)
                            heparin   tonics
                            horse serum   tranquilizers
                            iodides   vitamins
                            laxatives

Which infections are most apt to cause welts?
The most common would be bacterial infections located in the tonsils, adenoids, teeth, gums, sinuses, gall or urinary bladder, or lungs. Patients recovering from diseases such as scarlet fever, anthrax, brucellosis, or pseudomonas also may have welts. Other causes are virus, fungus (feet or body), spirochete (syphilis) or parasite (worm) infections.

Which miscellaneous substances cause welts?

Body Preparations   *Odours or Inhaled Substances*
creams   aerosols (bathroom and kitchen)
cosmetics   ammonia fumes
dyes or sprays (hair)   animal hair or dandruff

powders
mouth wash
toothpaste
nail polish
soaps or bubble bath
perfume
wave set

castor beans
cooking odours (eggs and fish)
cosmetics
flour
formaldehyde
insecticides
paint
sulphur dioxide

Touched Substances
animal hair (dandruff or saliva)
clothing dyes
feathers
foods
insects (beetles, butterflies,
   caterpillars, cocoons)
moths
plants
Portuguese man-of-war (jelly fish)
silk
wool

Others
chlorinated or water-softened water
dust
excess allergy extract dosage
insect bites, stings or scabies
moulds or yeast
mercury tooth fillings
pollens
pregnancy
premenses
any chemical insecticide, dye, wax,
   or mould on fresh fruits,
   vegetables or cheese

Which diseases are sometimes associated with welts?

amyloidosis
infectious mononucleosis
kidney disease
leukemia
liver disease
lupus erythematosis
malignancy (Hodgkin's)

multiple myeloma
Raynaud's disease
rheumatoid disease
Stevens-Johnson
thyrotoxicosis
ulcerative colitis
viral infections

How can you determine the cause of welts?

It is not easy to determine the cause of welts unless they occur immediately after some unusual contact. If welts are a frequent problem, the most rewarding way to determine the cause is to keep an hour-by-hour history of "everything" which is either eaten, swallowed or touched for a 12 to 24 hour period *prior to noticing the first welt*. Take a piece of paper and write down the time the first welt was noted. Attempt to remember as much as possible about what happened the previous hour, the hour before that etc. for several hours. Keep these records and call them the "bad days". If welts occur each day, it is due to a daily exposure. If welts occur infrequently, it is due to something which the individual rarely eats or is seldom near. On occasion welts are related to an excessive amount of something. For example, eating a little bit of chocolate might cause no welts, but if you ate a large amount of chocolate, such as children do on holidays, it might cause severe hives and swelling.

Make notations of the commercial brand names of possible causes of your welts. For example, one brand or type of aspirin, soup, or meat might cause welts while another may not. A spice or dye used in one preparation might not be in another. For this reason all records must be very detailed and specific.

If welts occur repeatedly it is extremely difficult to come to any conclusions unless detailed records are kept related to *the few hours before the onset of each nettle rash episode*. Records also should be kept of the foods eaten, activities engaged in, and ordinary daily contacts for several days when no welts are noted. These "good" day lists would indicate which substances were *not* related to the welts. By comparing the "good day" records for 24-hour periods when you have no welts, with the so called "bad" day lists, it should be possible to determine which substances or contacts could have caused the problems. See page 173 for more details.

If welts occur almost every day, the clues to the cause may be determined by studying records of very "good" days when you have *no* welts compared to very "bad" days when you have very severe welts. If you have a few welts every single day, it is extremely difficult to find the answers.

Once you think you know the cause of the welts, deliberate testing with that item should NOT be attempted, if the previous welt reaction was severe. It would be best if a physician helped confirm what you thought caused the welts. For example, aspirin can cause fatalities in some allergic individuals. Under certain circumstances, and in some individuals, it can be dangerous to take something which may cause welts.

It may be impossible to determine the cause of the welts in some patients. The above method, however, greatly increases the chances of finding the answer to this difficult problem. If you adopt the attitude that no one can find the cause, your negative attitude will surely help prevent anyone from finding the answer.

If welts are an extreme problem and everything has been tried, it sometimes helps if a patient is hospitalized and given only one food item for a day or two. Other items are gradually readded one at a time to find out which ones cause difficulty.

Are welts more common in women?

They seem to be, especially in middle-aged females. Some women tend repeatedly to have welts before, during or after their menstrual periods, during pregnancy, or during menopause. These welts are sometimes related to a drug or medicine used at that particular time, but sometimes the cause is unknown. In some unexplained way such welts seem to be possibly related to hormonal changes.

Another type of welt tends to occur mostly in young females, when they exercise or are emotionally upset. This is called cholinergic urticaria.

How should welts be treated?

1. Apply an anti-itch preparation to the affected skin.
2. Take an antihistamine by mouth to decrease the itch.
3. If a food or drug is causing the welts, it is important to eliminate it from the body as quickly as possible. One of the fastest ways to do this is to try to vomit by putting a finger down the throat. If this is unsuccessful, some drug should be taken to cause the bowels to move so the offending substance is eliminated from the body.
4. If welts are extremely severe, an injection of an antihistamine or adrenaline is helpful.

How dangerous are welts?

A person who has severe welts often looks disfigured and may be most uncomfortable but there is seldom great danger. When the swelling stops, the face and eyes will again appear perfectly normal. Welts generally affect the skin. Welts are dangerous when they affect the breathing passageway but fortunately, this seldom occurs. If there is swelling of the back of the tongue, hoarseness, or difficult breathing, immediate medical help should be secured and an antihistamine and drug to treat asthma should be taken if these are available.

Should normal activities be stopped if welts are a problem?

Although you may look peculiar because of welts, if you feel fine, there is no reason to stay away from work, school, or play. Activity which causes overheating or excitement could cause hives to worsen. A nettle rash is not contagious.

What causes welts to occur during infections?

Many factors cause welts when someone is ill. They could be non-specific and due to a temperature. Welts could be due to a drug which was taken because of infection, or could be due to the infection itself. Welt-like rashes, for example, are often associated with some childhood viral infections.

The usual treatment for welts during infections is to stop or replace most of the drugs a person is taking. If the welts disappear within a few hours and do not recur, it is assumed that one of the drugs which had been discontinued was the cause of the problem. Unless the suspected drug were needed very badly it would not be given again to that individual. Substitute drugs are often available and can be used. There is no way at the present time to accurately test for most drug allergies. Many patients (and physicians) are therefore unsure whether a certain drug is causing welts or not.

What are rare causes of welts or a nettle rash?

Heat, light, and cold can sometimes cause this type of reaction. If someone is allergic to cold, for example, it may be dangerous to drink cold liquids. A swim in cold water could cause a massive body swelling or so many welts that the blood pressure falls, the person becomes unconscious and drowns. Children have died under such circumstances in shallow cold water pools.

Welts due to the sun may be helped by a sun-screen preparation. Persons who have welts from sunlight may have no difficulty once they have a slight tan. Sun welts are easy to diagnose because they appear only in skin areas exposed to sunlight.

Can body swelling (angioedema) be hereditary?

There is one type found in some families which lack an essential body enzyme. It begins in childhood or young adulthood. Welts and itching are absent but marked swelling occurs often with abdominal pain. Trauma or injury can precipitate extremely dangerous swelling affecting the vocal cord area causing difficult breathing and even death.

A blood examination can confirm this deficiency which may be suspected because relatives have the problem. Treatment requires a physician.

How helpful is skin testing in diagnosing welts?

If welts occur only once and never again, the causative factor is not important. If, however, the welts are chronic, the best method of determining the cause would be a detailed history. Study of records of everything eaten or placed in the mouth, or any unfamiliar contacts might help. Skin tests are seldom of value in finding the source of the problem. At times they might give some insight if the welts were due to dust, pets, mould spores, pollens, stinging insects or certain drugs. Welts are a major challenge if the cause is not determined and eliminated. Sometimes the problem persists because it requires a great deal of time on the part of both the physician and the patient in an attempt to find the cause. Unless both are willing to spend the time, the answer may be puzzling and elusive. It must be admitted that in spite of all an allergist may do, no cause for this complaint may be found in some patients.

Does allergy injection therapy help eliminate welts?

Because the cause of welts are most frequently foods or drugs, allergy extract treatments are not helpful. If welts were caused by contact with pollens, mould spores, stinging insects, or dust, extract therapy might be beneficial.

CHAPTER SIX

Ear allergy

Which ear problems can be caused by allergies?

An allergy can cause skin problems affecting the outer ear (earlobe) or ear canal and other difficulties within the middle ear or inner ear. The middle ear extends from behind the eardrum through a cavity, the Eustachian tube, to the back portion of the nose. The bones which transmit sound to the inner ear are located behind the ear drum. One part of the inner ear is concerned with our sense of balance. On *rare* occasions this can be affected by food allergies in particular and cause dizziness. See page 189.

What is chronic serous or secretory otitis?

This problem is sometimes recurrent, especially in children. It causes an unnatural accumulation of fluid behind the eardrum. If for any reason air cannot pass easily from the nose through the Eustachian tube into the middle ear cavity, fluid forms. Normally the Eustachian tube opens intermittently when we swallow, yawn, or chew. Each time it opens, air can pass into the middle ear. Common causes of blockage of the nose opening for the Eustachian tube could be due to swollen tissues in that area (allergy or infection), or due to enlarged adenoids.

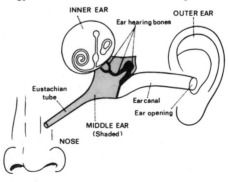

What are the symptoms of chronic secretory otitis?
There is often a mild or severe, intermittent or constant hearing loss. It is usually this hearing loss which causes the patient to be examined by an ear specialist. A feeling of fullness, blockage, popping, ringing, or crackling sounds may be evident. Pain or drainage from the ear may also be noted. Fever is seldom present. It is not uncommon for both ears to be affected although one is often worse than the other.

Some patients surprisingly have no obvious hearing loss. The problem is detected during a routine hearing test in school. Chronic secretory otitis is most common between the ages of about 3 and 10 years but it can sometimes also affect adults.

How is chronic secretory otitis treated?
The major purpose of all therapy is to allow the normal passage of air to and from the middle ear. This can be accomplished by keeping the nose end of the Eustachian tube patent or artificially by making an opening in the eardrum. If the cause of the fluid formation is an improperly functioning Eustachian tube, the obvious solution to the problem is to determine what is blocking the Eustachian tube or causing it to function improperly. If this causative factor can be eliminated, severe and permanent hearing problems can be prevented.

Most children who have middle ear fluid are helped by:

1. The judicious use of a combination of decongestants or antihistamines to decrease the swelling and secretions within that area. Nose drops are also helpful, in this regard.

2. By various methods which force air into the middle ear (ear popping). One method is to pinch the nose and to force air against the cheeks and mouth without allowing the cheeks to blow out. Ear popping helps if no nose infection is present.

3. By treating infection within the nose or sinuses that can cause swelling which blocks the opening of the Eustachian tubes. Antibiotics may help eliminate the infection and swelling.

4. By surgically removing enlarged or infected adenoids to relieve their ear problems.

5. Others are helped by placing a tiny open plastic tube through the eardrum.

If the above measures need to be carried out repeatedly, it could indicate that allergy might possibly be a factor related to the problem. This would be true especially if the patient had other forms of allergies.

Why do tubes in eardrums help?
If the nose end of the Eustachian tube is blocked, air can enter the area behind the eardrum or middle ear if small open tubes are placed through the eardrums. By allowing air to easily pass into the middle ear, forma-

tion of fluid can be prevented and the tissues in that area can become more normal. In many patients, this form of management is very successful.

An ear surgeon may remove fluid from the middle ear through the small opening he makes when a tube is to be placed through the eardrum. This hole placed in the eardrum is called a myringotomy. The fluid is very difficult to remove because it can be unbelievably thick and viscous. Artificial eardrum openings tend to close quickly. Because of this, plastic open tubes are placed through the hole in the eardrum so it remains open.

Eardrum tubes usually fall out or sometimes are removed by the ear surgeon after several (6 to 12) months. In most patients the problems have resolved themselves after that period of time because the swollen tissues, which originally caused obstruction of the Eustachian tube, have returned to normal. Air can now easily enter through the nose opening of the Eustachian tube and an artificial opening in the eardrum no longer is necessary. In a few patients however, when the tiny air tube is no longer in the eardrum, the process begins again and fluid re-forms behind the drum causing hearing loss.

It is sometimes necessary to replace eardrum tubes repeatedly to maintain air in the middle ear cavity. If fluid is allowed to remain in the middle ear, it can cause the little hearing bones which are located behind the eardrums to stick together or be cemented so that sound cannot be sent normally to the inner ear. This sometimes causes permanent hearing loss.

Do ear tubes damage eardrums?

In many patients repeated insertion of ear tubes has not caused any permanent damage to the eardrum. This procedure does, however, tend to cause the drums to become thin and eventually the drums may no longer be able to retain or hold the plastic tubes.

What are the major disadvantages of ear tubes?

The major problem is that a patient usually has to have a general anaesthetic at the time of each tube insertion. If there are openings in the eardrums it is difficult to wash a child's hair or to allow swimming. Some ear physicians allow some patients to use greased knitting wool ear plugs and tight fitting bathing caps but others do not feel swimming is advisable under any circumstance. Diving is definitely not permitted for persons who have tubes within their ears.

Who is most likely to have allergic ear problems?

These are most apt to occur in patients who:
1.   Have other allergies or allergic parents or relatives.

2.   Have allergies each year at the same time possibly caused by certain pollens or mould spores.
3.   Have an excessive number of eosinophils within their blood, nose mucus, or ear fluid. This type of white blood cell (eosinophil) is often found in excess in allergic patients.
4.   Have positive skin reactions to common allergenic substances.
5.   Repeatedly have had their tonsils or adenoids removed or needed this operation prior to the age of 3 years.
6.   Have had to have ear tubes *repeatedly* placed in the eardrums.

Which allergenic substances cause ear allergies?
The most frequent ones are dust, moulds, feathers, pets, kapok, and foods such as milk, corn, peanuts, wheat, eggs, chicken and chocolate. Exposure to cats, feathers, or certain foods sometimes can cause a sudden occurrence of ear fluid and symptoms.

Are allergy skin tests helpful for ear patients?
Skin test reactions in patients who have ear problems due to allergies are sometimes less strong, less numerous, and less reliable than they are in hay fever or asthma patients.

How would an allergy affecting the middle ear be treated?
If allergic swelling of nose tissue blocks the opening of the Eustachian tube, it is possible that antihistamines, decongestants, or nose drops or other nose drugs may temporarily help. In some patients, ear symptoms can be relieved on a relatively permanent basis if their home is made allergy-free. (See Chapter 11).
Other children find relief by eliminating certain foods or by trying diets. This would be helpful only if a food were the cause of the nose or middle ear tissue swelling. (See Chapter 12).
Some children improve if they receive allergy extract injection therapy after skin testing. In summary many patients who have hearing problems on an allergic basis respond to one or some combination of
1.   allergy control within their home
2.   diet changes
3.   allergy extract therapy.

How can you determine a hearing loss?
The most accurate method would be to have a hearing test or audiogram done. The following might indicate the need for this test:
1.   Although children may not hear when it is time to do household chores or to go to bed, it is significant if they do not hear when they are called about something which interests them greatly, i.e. dessert.
2.   Children and adults who cannot hear well, often tend to speak

louder than normal. It may not be an indication of a hearing problem if a
person plays music or listens to television which is much too loud.

   3.   Sometimes a youngster will answer a phone and state no one has
called as he hangs up. If your friends complain that this happens it could
be that the child does not hear the caller's voice.

   4.   Have your youngster shut his eyes and place a ticking watch very
close to one ear. If the youngster can hear it on one side but repeatedly
cannot hear it on the other side, this might indicate a hearing loss.

Can you help your physician detect a hearing loss?

   Physicians can obtain much information about a person's hearing by
doing tuning fork tests. In order to do these tests, a youngster must be
able to tell the difference between loud and soft. A parent can teach a
youngster what these two words mean by playing a game of making two
sounds and having the youngster tell which is louder and which is softer.
It will then be much easier when the youngster is asked by the physician
to tell whether a sound is louder in front or behind his ear. The youngster
should be told to tell the doctor if he does not hear any sound at all.
Children are confused if asked to compare two sounds when they hear
only one.

How significant is a poor hearing test?

   There are many causes for a poor hearing test in school. One of the
most common is that the youngster has a nose cold or infection which has
caused temporary nose tissue swelling. A subsequent hearing test might
reveal normal hearing. Allergy nose swelling, however, can cause a
temporary hearing loss if exposure to the allergenic substance is intermittent. Sometimes children have a poor hearing test because of excess
ear wax in the ear canal. Quite often hearing tests are unreliable because
a child is confused about what he is to do or say.

How can a hearing loss affect schoolwork?

   A hearing loss, even if it is minimal, can cause major problems in a
school situation where it is so important to hear directions properly.
Minimal hearing losses are difficult for parents to detect and children
may not know that they do not hear properly. Alert school teachers
or routine hearing tests are helpful in detecting hearing loss in some
children.

How can schoolwork be improved if there is a one-sided hearing loss?

   If a child hears best on one side, be sure the child sits in the classroom
so that most of the sound from the teacher is directed towards the "good"
ear. For example, if a child hears best with the right ear, he should be

sitting on the left side of the room so that the teacher's voice is directed towards the right ear.

Do allergies influence the indications for tonsil or adenoid removal?
The recommendations for tonsillectomy and adenoidectomy are similar for allergic and non allergic children and adults. A person, however, who has hay fever should not have his tonsils and adenoids removed during a pollen season (See page 53 for your area). Asthma sometimes may begin for the first time if this is done. Any nose or throat surgery can sometimes cause severe asthma in adults who have nose polyps. (See page 212). Many children's hearing problems disappear if their tonsils and adenoids are removed. If hearing is not restored, an allergist might be helpful.

What are frequent indications for removal of tonsils and adenoids?
1.   Repeated severe infections of the tonsils or adenoids.
2.   Difficulty swallowing because of large tonsils or noisy difficult breathing because of markedly enlarged adenoids. Tonsils and adenoids normally increase in size until the age of ten years before they tend to become much smaller. One should therefore seriously consider the necessity of removing these tissues because of their size if nature will solve the problem within a relatively short period of time.
3.   A localized area of pus behind or around the tonsils (a tonsillar abscess).
4.   Recurrent or permanent hearing loss.
5.   Abnormalities in dentition due to mouth breathing. Enlarged adenoids may prevent normal breathing through the nose. The final decision about any person's adenoids and tonsils should depend not only upon the opinion of the family physician or pediatrician but also upon that of the ear, nose and throat specialist (otolaryngologist).
There are some parents who seem to be unusually anxious to have tonsils and adenoids removed in all their children. These tissues, may not be essential, but they are functional and should be removed only when necessary.

Can dizziness or vertigo be on an allergic basis?
The most common cause of this type of problem is certainly not allergies but in some allergic adults or children foods, in particular, can cause an alteration in their sense of balance. This may be associated with buzzing noises, a feeling of the ears being blocked, intestinal upsets such as nausea or vomiting, emotional upsets, or fatigue. (See Chapter 8).

CHAPTER SEVEN

Special infant allergy problems

What types of allergies do infants have?

1. Allergy often first appears in the form of a cheek rash sometime during the first 6 months, and as time passes the rash will be found mainly in front of the elbows and in back of the knees or around the wrists, ankles and calves. This rash is called eczema or atopic dermatitis. (See Chapter 4). Nettle rash or welts can also appear.

2. Intestinal allergies are commonly seen in infants. Young babies without allergies may have colic during the first 3 to 6 months of life but allergic infants may have this problem for the entire first year of life or longer. Colicky infants pull their legs on their bellies and cry with discomfort. They appear hungry but are obviously very uncomfortable after eating. When this problem persists beyond 3 to 6 months, it may indicate a food allergy. Allergic babies also may have excessive gas which is passed rectally or by mouth, excess mucus in their bowel movements, diarrhoea or soft stools, spitting up, and painful mouth ulcers (canker sores). A most frequent cause of allergic bowel problems is either milk or cereal. Any baby who does not seem better when his formula is changed frequently may have a food allergy. (See Chapter 12 related to food allergies).

3. Nose allergies can occur in infants. This allergy is characterized by a watery drippy nose, stuffiness and difficulty breathing through the nose. (See Chapter 2). Many parents are perplexed because their infant has a constant "cold" but does not seem ill. The infant has, in fact, nose allergies. These infants have difficulty taking their formula because they cannot breathe and suck at the same time. They therefore suck vigorously for a short while, push the nipple out of their mouth, and then breathe quickly. They repeatedly do this during each feeding.

4. Irritability and restlessness are not uncommon in allergic infants. Frequently they cannot rest at night or sleep 8 hours. When the allergenic factor is eliminated, they sleep well and are obviously happier and more content.

5. Infants who have chest allergies frequently cough and may have difficulty not only breathing out, but breathing in. A chest rattle or squeak may be heard as they breathe. Unlike older children and adults, infants can lie flat when they are in severe respiratory distress.

6. Recurrent infections may sometimes be a problem in allergic infants. Allergically swollen tissues seem to be more prone to infection. Once the allergies are treated, germs invade less readily and the blood supply improves. This may help to decrease the tendency to infection.

It must be remembered that although all of the above symptoms can be due to allergies, they also can be caused by many other medical problems. It is absolutely essential that your infant be examined by your physician before any diagnosis is made. For example bronchiolitis, which is a viral infection of infancy, definitely can cause wheezing. It is difficult to tell the difference between asthma and this disease. It is significant that many children or adults who later develop asthma have a history of having had bronchiolitis in infancy.

Which foods are most apt to cause infant allergies?
Milk, cereals (wheat in particular), eggs, chicken, and any foods which contain any of these items are major offenders. Some allergists have advised eggs not be given for the first 12 months and that wheat and chicken be withheld for at least 9 months. These precautions possibly reduce the tendency to develop skin, chest and nose allergies in the allergy-prone infant. The major cause of any allergic symptom in an infant under the age of 1 year is a food.

It is not understood or readily explained but if a food causes an infant's symptoms, merely omitting it from the diet for a period of several weeks or months may eliminate the allergy. After that period of time eating the food does not seem to cause allergies, as it once did. This would be true for only some food allergies, which were not extreme.

Although soya bean milk and rice are generally considered not to cause allergies, under certain circumstances these foods can cause allergy. It is possible for example to be placed on soya bean "milk" and to develop an allergy to this, instead of to cow's milk. Cow's milk is more allergenic, however, than soya milk.

On page 163 there is a list of the most and least allergenic foods. In a particular patient, this list might not be applicable, but in general, it should prove helpful. It must be understood even though some food causes a symptom, it is not necessarily due to an allergy. (See page 189 concerning other causes of difficulties associated with eating certain foods.)

Can babies have a natural aversion to foods causing allergy?
Although an infant might refuse to eat a food to which he is sensitive, it

is possible he may have an unusual liking for it. Rice, wheat, and oat cereal, for example, can sometimes cause almost a compulsive type of eating, even though they may cause abdominal pain. Because the baby likes the food and acts hungry, his mother gives that food repeatedly and a vicious circle is started.

Infants who are very allergic to eggs or fish, even if a few months old, will often refuse these foods. The food may cause an immediate reaction in the mouth to which even a very young baby will react. Trying to force a baby to take a teaspoon of the food which he cannot tolerate can cause immediate and dangerous symptoms. If this food is swallowed, sudden vomiting followed by diarrhoea can occur. The lips, face, or throat can swell causing great difficulty in breathing.

Which meats are least allergenic in the infant period?

Lamb is the least, while chicken and pork are most allergenic. Beef may or may not cause difficulty. Some allergic patients have symptoms from eggs and also from female chicken, while eating a male cockerel or capon causes no difficulty. We cannot adequately explain this.

Can a parent detect an infant food allergy?

Although parents can observe their infant, because growth occurs so quickly, it is essential to have a physician's supervision while trying to detect a food allergy.

If a parent suspects only one food of causing a mild allergy, that food should be omitted *in all forms* (See page 172) for a minimum of at least 14 days. Within 2 weeks, or earlier if the infant improves more rapidly, the food can be eaten again. If the omitted food caused allergies, the symptoms should stop when the food isn't eaten and should recur and become progressively more severe when the food is eaten again. Any food can be checked in the manner just outlined but this should not be done if a food causes obvious serious symptoms as soon as an infant eats it. If food allergic symptoms occur each day, it must be due to a food eaten every day. If, however, food symptoms occur infrequently it must be a food that is seldom eaten. (See page 172 for information to help detect the cause of this type of allergy).

Symptoms from foods often do not occur on the day when they are eaten but on the day after or even later. Under these circumstances, it can be most difficult to determine food allergies and a physician's aid would be required.

If a parent suspects several foods it can prove to be much more difficult than determining a single food allergy. Suppose an infant is allergic to milk, wheat and eggs. When you introduce wheat, it may be difficult to notice any increase of symptoms because the baby has had daily difficulty. Unless you eliminate most or all of the allergenic foods all at once;

it is hard to detect the cause of a food allergy.

The following diet is helpful for infants under 1 year. In general select 2 or 3 cereals, vegetables or fruits in each category, providing the baby *seldom* eats these particular items. Do *not* select frequently eaten foods.

SPECIAL DIET FOR INFANTS

soya bean milk and kosher milk-free margarine
rice, barley, oats, or rye cereal
carrots, string beans, squash, sweet potatoes
applesauce, pears, peaches, apricots and their juices
chicken (capon or rooster) or lamb
salt, sugar, and water
water-soluble vitamins A, D, and C.

Your infant should be kept on this diet until he seems to improve but never more than 14 days. If the diet is helpful, improvement is often noted in less than 5 days but sometimes it may take 10 to 14 days. If there is no improvement after this period it could indicate there was no food allergy or the infant was allergic to some food included in the two week diet. It is possible that more prolonged or complicated dietary study is needed for some infants but a medical specialist's help would be essential.

If an infant did improve during the 2 week diet, it would indicate that allergenic foods had been eliminated. Suggestions concerning how to re-add foods to determine which might be causing the allergy is discussed on pages 172 to 180.

What problems arise when parents try diet studies?

1. A common error is for parents not to read food labels thoroughly. Many are not aware that milk and wheat can be found in soups, or eggs in mayonnaise, or milk in bread and margarine. See page 180.

2. Parents may not understand that a speck of a food can cause allergy symptoms. See page 166. It is possible to do dietary studies on and off for years and never detect the true cause of the food allergies because someone always makes a mistake and gives the baby a little bit of food that wasn't supposed to be eaten.

3. Persons concerned with diet studies become discouraged when improvement is not immediate. Parents must be patient. The diet must be carried out long enough so that a decision can be made in one direction or the other regarding allergies.

4. Infections may complicate the interpretation of diet studies See page 169.

5. Infants grow so rapidly, it is essential that calcium supplements be

added to their diet if milk is omitted for more than 2 weeks. See page 184 Your physician will advise you. If the baby drinks enough soya bean milk, there is no problem in relation to the calcium or bone growth. See page 183.

6. When doing dietary studies, unsuspected allergies may be detected. For example a parent may want to watch the effect of a diet upon the skin. The skin might not improve, but a parent might notice irritability, belly ache, stuffy nose, or night restlessness disappears during the special diet and these problems recur when a normal diet is resumed. Further study may detect the exact cause of the baby's symptoms.

7. Parents may find a food such as wheat eliminates their infant's symptoms, but be reluctant to admit it because they do not want to omit this food from the baby's diet. The allergy often persists until the cause is eliminated, even if it is difficult to avoid wheat (flour) products, for example.

Should vitamins be given during infant diet studies?

Infants grow so quickly that vitamins should not be discontinued for more than 10 to 14 days at any time during the first 9 months of life. Vitamins should be readded to the basic diet for a period of 3 days as a single food as suggested on page 172. If you suspect that your infant has a vitamin allergy, see page 180.

What special substances cause infant allergies?

Adult and children's allergies may be due to many similar substances such as dust or pets (see page 191) but babies have some special exposures which can cause difficulty. The use of perfumed body powders, oils, lotions, soap, scented diapers, and diaper cleaning agents can cause symptoms. It may be necessary to avoid scented facial or toilet tissue or nice-smelling aerosols in the bathroom or kitchen.

Parents frequently use vaporizers or humidifiers in their bedrooms. These can become contaminated with moulds or bacteria and cause symptoms. (See page 155).

Animal hair, dandruff, or saliva can cause difficulty. It is possible for a baby's stuffed toy or playpen pad or mattress to have animal hair in them. A baby's mattress should be synthetic or covered entirely by plastic and stuffed toys must be allergy-free both inside and outside.

Woollen or fuzzy blankets or wool covered furniture can cause symptoms. Infants can have difficulty when they are held by someone wearing woollen clothing.

Parents should be extremely careful to keep their infant's bedroom entirely allergy-free and allow their baby to nap only in his own room. Allergic infants should not be exposed to feather pillows, woollen blankets, and allergenic mattresses.

Can infant allergies be prevented?

An attempt can certainly be made in this direction.

a. The bedroom should be kept as free of allergenic substances as possible and an effort must be made to keep the infant away from highly allergenic substances. (See page 85 and Chapter 11).

b. Parents must avoid acquiring any pet which has fur or feathers.

c. Foods should be added singly and slowly during infancy. It is best to breast feed an infant since allergy to breast milk is rare. When breast feeding is impossible, many allergists recommend the use of soya bean milk although the evidence that this prevents allergy is not without controversy. As new foods are added to the baby's diet, small amounts should be given on the first day and gradually increasing amounts thereafter.

Fruits and vegetables, should be given individually at first and not in mixtures until all components of the mixture have been checked. A definite attempt must be made to delay the addition of highly allergenic foods such as eggs, chocolate, nuts, peanut butter and fish. The excessive use of wheat products or orange juice is also to be discouraged.

d. Potentially allergic children should be given synthetic vitamins. Cod liver oil preparations should never be given to anyone known to have a fish allergy.

It is possible for the flavour or colour of a vitamin preparation to cause allergic symptoms. (See page 180 for aid to detect a vitamin allergy).

e. Stuffed animals or toys should be thoroughly examined both inside and outside to see if they contain any allergenic substance. They also should be washable and cleaned at least monthly. (See page 11 and Chapter 1).

f. Extremely allergic infants may develop pollen and mould spore symptoms by the age of 2 or 3 years. By installing either a room or furnace air purifying system, some allergists believe that a sensitivity to these new substances might be delayed or prevented. (See pages 151 to 156).

g. Parents must be extremely careful if an infant has diarrhoea not to feed highly allergenic foods until the bowels are normal again. (See page 163). Shortly after a belly upset, the intestines are more porous or open than normal and sensitivity to a highly allergenic food eaten during that period can more easily develop.

Is it possible for an infant to outgrow his allergies?

An allergic infant is in a state of flux. He may tend to "lose" one symptom only to acquire another. For example, food allergies which could cause eczema or intestinal problems tend to disappear by the time the infant is 1 to 3 years of age. Then, however, other forms of allergies may develop such as nose or chest symptoms due to dust, wool, pets, or moulds. Pollen sensitivities usually do not appear until a child is at least 2 or 3 years old. Occasionally, however, an infant can have symptoms due to pollen before the age of two years. Any of these later allergies may be "outgrown" or last for years. (See page 13).

Should potentially allergic infants be breast fed?

Breast-fed babies have potentially fewer allergies and grow well. Although foods and drugs which mother eats can pass through the milk, there is no doubt that breast milk is less allergenic than cow's milk. If breast milk seems to be causing symptoms, elimination of highly allergenic foods from the mother's diet will often solve the problem.

Can a pregnant woman's diet affect her unborn baby?

There is controversy concerning which diets are best for mothers to help prevent infant allergies. A widely varied diet is often recommended which avoids excessive amounts of highly allergenic foods. The pregnant woman should be certain that she eats the proper foods, and takes the correct vitamins and minerals to assure normal growth of her developing baby.

Should all potentially allergic babies be fed soya bean milk?

Unfortunately the evidence that this is either beneficial or necessary is not clear. It might make a baby become allergic to soya bean milk rather than cow's milk. Cow's milk allergy may be more common because more babies drink it. If, however, every effort is to be taken to avoid allergies in an infant, that baby should be breast fed. If this is impossible, some allergists would advise that soya bean milk be used. This recommendation may mean that many potentially allergic infants are fed soya bean milk needlessly. Even if an allergy to soya bean milk develops, it is easier to avoid soya bean products, than it is to avoid milk.

One disadvantage in relation to soya bean milk is that it costs more than milk. Most infants drink 1 to 2 cans of soya milk per day. Soya bean or milk fed babies grow equally well.

Is the milk of goats or cows less allergenic?

Any form of animal milk can cause allergies. It is the protein part of the milk which causes symptoms. Sour milk separates into the cottage cheese or the casein part and a clear liquid portion called whey. The casein milk protein of all animals is so similar that someone allergic to cow's casein, also probably would be allergic to goat's casein. Several different proteins in the whey part of milk can cause allergy. It is possible to be allergic to a protein in cow whey which is unlike that protein in goat's whey. In this rare situation, goat's milk might not cause symptoms while cow's milk would.

Are milk substitutes available for babies?
There are some milk substitutes which are entirely unrelated to milk. For example, soya bean milk is not milk, it is really a bean soup. There are also some types of meat soups which are called "milk". All these preparations should supply proteins which infants need and usually obtain from milk but check with your doctor.

Which fruits or juices are least allergenic?
Pear, peach, apricot, plum and pineapple supposedly cause few allergies. Pears, however, on occasion have caused a rash in some babies. Berries are not considered to be very allergenic during the infant period. Citrus fruits (i.e. orange) and bananas sometimes can cause infant allergy.

Which vegetables are least apt to cause infant allergies?
The least allergenic are beets, carrots, squash, string beans and sweet potatoes. The most allergenic are peas, corn, tomatoes, and white potatoes. Exceptions, of course, can occur.

Which cereals cause few allergies?
The cereal which an infant eats least is usually the one which will not cause allergies. Since many infants eat wheat, this is often a cause of allergy. In general, rice, barley, and oats are less allergenic. Any baby, however, can become allergic to any cereal and some babies are allergic to all cereals. Some allergists recommend poi cereal of the type eaten in Hawaii. This, however, is not available in most countries.

At what age should an infant see an allergist?
An allergist should be contacted if an infant is extremely uncomfortable or seems unwell because of an allergy. Parents may be reluctant to see a specialist because they believe that their baby will have to have allergy skin tests and extract treatment. Foods are the major cause of an infant's allergies and are best studied by diets. The other major cause of allergies in infancy is related to home. (See page 139 and Chapter 11). Only the exceptional infant would have to be skin tested and these allergy tests would not be numerous or particularly difficult to do. The major reason for seeing an allergist, if one is available, is not only to determine the cause of the present difficulty but to help prevent future allergies from developing.

Is it ever necessary to give injection treatments to infants?
Some allergists never give extract therapy for allergy during infancy. Others believe that in selected patients, it might be indicated if a baby had severe allergies which did not respond to dietary management and home changes.

CHAPTER EIGHT

Possible uncommon forms of allergy

There are some medical problems which have been attributed to allergy which have caused much controversy among allergists. Many believe that these problems are not due to allergy while others are convinced that allergies are a factor in *some* patients. A few of these will be mentioned. With research and time, more understanding of their true relation to allergy should be known.

What possible nervous system allergies have been described?

These would include various types of headaches, epilepsy, tension, nervousness, emotional problems, and strange body swelling.

Which foods have been thought possibly to trigger epilepsy?

It has been reported by a few allergists that milk (cheese), eggs, wheat, or chocolate could be related to this problem in some patients.

Can asthmatics have epilepsy associated only with their attacks?

Yes, this can occur but the convulsions are not due to exposure to an allergenic substance. The seizures are believed to be caused by asthma. Some patients have changes in their brainwave or electroencephalogram.

What is a migraine?

Migraine headaches occur periodically, are one-sided, and may be preceded by some visual disturbance or digestive problem. The headache may be throbbing and pulsating, and completely incapacitate an individual. They occur more often in females and are much more common after puberty. Migraine may be more common in allergic families but this has not been adequately proven.

Which warning symptoms may precede a migraine attack?

The indications that a headache may begin in a few hours vary among individuals. Some notice weakness, feel especially tired, look pale, seem upset or depressed, see strange lights, or have changes in their vision which can cause them to prefer darkness. Nausea is often present. The headaches may occur suddenly or develop gradually.

What triggers migraine headaches?

Foods such as chocolate, cheese, milk, wheat, and eggs commonly cause this problem in some persons. Alcohol has also been related to some attacks. Excitement, irritating odours (smoke), emotional upsets, and adverse weather conditions sometimes also precipitate attacks. Attacks may occur immediately or several hours after exposure to the offending substance.

There is evidence to show that in some persons this type of headache may be due to an enzyme disturbance. Certain foods, for example cheese and chocolate, may require a specific enzyme for digestion. If the enzyme is lacking, chemicals produced by altered food digestion cause the headache. Patients often assume the problem is due to a food allergy. It is not. See pages 156 – 190

Sometimes these headaches are first noted when menstrual periods begin and disappear after menopause for reasons which are not easily explained. Headaches have also occurred in association with the use of oral contraceptives. Hormones seem to be related to some such headaches. Women who gain a large amount of fluid weight in association with their menses or ovulation are particularly prone to migraine. This type may be helped with estrogens and diuretics.

How long does a migraine headache last?

A typical attack may last a few hours or may continue for several days. Occasionally, attacks may last only a few minutes.

What is a histamine or Horton's headache?

There is one special type which is called a histamine headache (Horton's). This occurs mainly in men, appears suddenly, lasts for hours to days and then rapidly disappears. The next episode may occur again after a short or long period of time. Patients with this problem typically have a headache, a runny watery eye, and nose symptoms ONLY on one side of the face. There are many variations and sometimes one symptom will overshadow the rest. Some persons have abdominal discomfort and lack the headache, although they have one-sided nose and eye symptoms. Patients often falsely believe themselves to be allergic because their "hay fever-like" symptoms are so severe. A number of drugs are often helpful but some patients respond poorly to any form of treatment.

Can allergy cause dizziness?
Some physicians believe that some patients who have dizziness in association with Meniere's disease have food allergy, especially to milk. Studies to confirm or deny this are presently being carried out.

Can allergy cause bed wetting?
This has been said to be caused by milk, tomato, citrus fruits and flavourings, food colours, and black pepper. If this problem is caused by allergy, it is most uncommon.

What is a chemically intolerant person?
There are a few persons who believe themselves to be sensitive to odours of oil, gas, chemicals, and construction materials used in building a home. See table 1. These people may claim they can sometimes detect which items used in home construction cause difficulty by merely sniffing them. Possible factors would include tar paper, cement or rubber sealers, asphalt, wood preservatives, adhesives, silicone sealers, various types of rubber products, plastic vinyl, wall or roof sheeting insulation such as rock wool, wallpaper pastes, wall and floor coverings or materials, caulking compounds, termite infested dirt fill, odorous woods such as cedar or redwood paints.

Which unusual items might trigger allergic symptoms?

276   Special Aids to Help Parents

ODOURS WHICH CAN TRIGGER ALLERGIC SYMPTOMS*

adhesive tape	grease
aerosols	hair preparations
alcohol (rubbing)	incense
ammonia	ink, marking pens
banana oil	insect repellents (spray or
bleaches, chlorine type	candles)
bubble bath or oils	moth balls
buckwheat flour	paints, paint thinners, varnishes,
burning wood, pine cones,	lacquer, shellac
candles, paper, trash	paper (news, ditto, carbon,
camphor	mimeograph)
castor beans (flour or oil)	perfumes
Christmas trees or decorations	plastic containers, cements
cleaning fluid for clothing	polish for fingernails, metal,
or windows	shoes, or furniture

coal, gasoline, kerosene, oil, wood
cosmetics
cooking, especially fish or eggs or flour dust
creosote
chlorinated water
deodorants
detergents
disinfectants
dyes for cloth, cosmetics, or shoes
exterminating compounds
floor wax
frying foods
fumes from exhaust, garage, garbage, or factory
gas from leaky stove or refrigerator
polyurethane
phenol products (Lysol)
rubber bedding, paints or its sanding or woodwork
scented facial and toilet tissue
smoke from any source, including cigarettes
soaps
sulphur dioxide
tar fumes, or tar-based shampoos and ointments
tobacco
turpentine
typewriter-ribbons or stencils
vegetables while cooking such as onions, peas, beans, cabbages and potatoes
wood— cedar or pine

* From Theron Randolph, *Human Ecology and Susceptibility to the Chemical Environment, 1967,* Charles C Thomas, Publisher, Springfield, Illinois. Used by permission.

Miscellaneous

UNUSUAL ITEMS WHICH MAY BE RESPONSIBLE FOR ALLERGIC SYMPTOMS*

air-conditioning
antibiotics, hormones, or preservatives in or on foods
artificial food colourings
artificial sweeteners
braces for teeth
clothes starch
cornstarch
cosmetics
dyes in medicines
fillings in teeth
mouthwash
nylon in any form
hair dyes and permanent waving
plastics in any form (plastic home-made toys)

rayon or cellulose clothing
shoe polish
toothpastes
Vaseline and petroleum products
water (softened, chlorinated, fluoridated)
waxes on fruits and vegetables

* From Theron Randolph, *Human Ecology and Susceptibility to the Chemical Environment*, 1967, Charles C Thomas, Publisher, Springfield, Illinois. Used by permission.

CHAPTER NINE

Drugs which help allergies

GENERALITIES CONCERNING DRUGS

When should you take a drug?

Drugs should be taken whenever a medical problem or symptom is severe enough to interfere with normal activities. Every slight headache may not require aspirin, but if the headache is severe or persistent, you should take medication. A few coughs probably won't require treatment, but if it persists, drugs might be helpful.

When should you stop taking drugs?

This depends entirely upon why the drug was taken and who ordered it. For example, if your headache disappears after an aspirin, you don't need more aspirin. Your physician may recommend an antibiotic for a certain number of days to treat an infection. You must be extremely careful to take the treatment for the *full* period of time specified by your doctor. You may feel better in a day or two, but the antibiotic should be continued for as long a period of time as recommended by your doctor. (See page 115).

Many infections are caused by germs, most often bacteria, viruses, or fungi (yeasts). Sometimes after being treated for a bacterial infection, body fungi become a problem causing a fungus infection which needs to be treated. Women in particular note this problem. A vaginal discharge due to an abundance of a fungus can develop which requires treatment with a special antibiotic. Sometimes males and females develop an itchy rectal or anal area, which they do not realize is a common complication after the use of an antibiotic. The overgrowth of yeasts and moulds caused by antibiotics can also sometimes cause an inflamed throat or diarrhoea.

Is it important to give drugs several times daily?

Many drugs are supposed to be given 3 or 4 times a day, which means they should be taken every 4 to 6 hours. Some drugs are long acting and taken only once or twice a day. At the beginning of a severe infection, your physician may recommend antibiotics be given every 6 hours day and night. This may bring an infection under control earlier.

Always give the drugs at the interval suggested by your doctor, so that the drug blood level remains high. If the antibiotic blood level falls because the drug is overdue by a few hours, germs can multiply and this would prolong infection. When you swallow a drug, it probably is absorbed from the stomach into your blood. The blood level gradually rises to a certain level and falls slightly over a period of hours. The aim of giving drugs at regular intervals is to keep the blood level high enough so that offending germs can't multiply or are killed.

How often should drugs be taken?

Prescriptions may state that drugs should be taken, for example, every 6 hours. This would mean, for example, that if the first dose was taken at 8.30 a.m., repeat it at 2.30 p.m., 8.30 p.m., and at 2.30 a.m. If you wonder if the drug should be given in the middle of the night, check with your physician.

It is common for prescriptions to be labelled to take a drug 3 or 4 times a day. This means you should divide the waking hours by 3 or 4 and take the drugs at that particular interval. For example, if you arise at 8 a.m., and retire at 11 p.m., then it means that the medicine should be taken at 8.00 a.m., 1.00 p.m., 6.00 p.m., and 11.00 p.m. If drugs are to be given 3 times a day and a child arises and retires at 8.00 o'clock, give the drug at 8.00 a.m., 2.00 p.m., and 8.00 p.m.

When should drugs be given during sleep?

This might be required if an individual were extremely ill, for example, early in the treatment of an infection.

In general, it is unwise to awaken a patient who is not in distress and who is sleeping well. If an asthmatic is sleeping quietly and in no respiratory distress, he needs no drugs during the night. If, however, a patient is struggling to breathe and wheezing, he should be awakened and given the appropriate drugs. Also give a large glass of water to help thin the mucus.

How soon does a drug help after it has been taken?

In general, liquid medicines help more quickly than tablet forms. Most swallowed drugs start to help in about 20 minutes. Chewable tablets should be well-chewed because this will speed their absorption. Rectal liquid medicine is often quickly absorbed but this is not true for rectal suppositories. Sometimes these help in a ½ hour, but it might take hours before any benefit would be noticed. Drugs placed under the tongue (sublingual) usually help in a few seconds.

Asthma is sometimes treated by sprays which helps medicine to pass from the mouth to the lungs. Relief can occur quickly and lasts from 20 minutes to several hours depending upon the type used. With severe asthma, if a spray is used again and again, it not only may not help but it can be harmful and definitely make asthma worse in some patients.

The major advantage of spray drugs is that some wheezing episodes can be quickly stopped. For example, night coughs which often precede severe wheezing may stop immediately thus preventing asthma if a spray is used. See page 107 for more information about sprays.

How long do drugs act?

Drugs help for different lengths of time. Drugs given every 4 to 6 hours will probably last about that long. Long-acting drugs supposedly relieve a patient's symptoms for 8 to 12 hours. Many long-acting drugs, however, do not help as long as they should. For this reason, 4-hour drugs are generally preferable except at bedtime.

If a 4 to 6 hour drug helps for 2 hours, do not take the drug every two hours because this might cause poisoning or bad reactions. Discuss such problems with your physician.

What should you do if a drug doesn't help?

Check with your physician. Sometimes drugs don't help because it may take hours or days before their effect would be noticed. Sometimes they don't help because they are taken or used incorrectly.

Surprising studies of drug use have shown that patients *seldom* take treatment exactly as it has been prescribed and for the period of time suggested by the physician. This accounts for many poor responses to drugs.

How can you decide which of several drugs to use?

Take one drug, for example to treat hay fever, and notice whether it helps within a ½ hour or so. If that medicine does not seem to help in any way, you should not try another sample drug until the potential effect of the first drug is gone. In other words, if it was supposed to be taken three times a day, you should not try another drug for 4 hours. Continue to check other drugs in the same manner until you find an effective one.

Allergic persons must be careful not to take several similar drugs such as more than one antihistamine at one time. This would be similar to using different brands of aspirin all at once, and could cause overdosage and illness because too much was taken. Your physician will tell you when it is safe to use several drugs at the same time.

What should you do if a drug helps but causes some undesirable effect?

This is not uncommon. Antibiotics may help to eliminate infection but can cause diarrhoea. Asthma drugs can relieve asthma but make patients very nervous or cause an upset stomach. Drugs for nose allergy may cause drowsiness. Discuss such problems with your doctor.

Can a drug cause an allergy?

Drugs certainly do cause allergies. The main ingredient can cause symptoms but patients can be allergic also to certain colours or flavours used in drugs or medicines. Persons allergic to corn syrup or alcohol may have difficulty from medicine which contains these items. Some people are allergic to a binder which helps medical powders stick together so they can be pressed into pill shapes.

Should a patient take several drugs at the same time?

Under certain circumstances several different drugs can safely be taken at the same time when these are being used to help different symptoms. For example, if a person has asthma, nose allergies, a fever, and an infection, he can take simultaneously a medicine to treat asthma, an antihistamine, asprin, and an antibiotic. When using several drugs, however, always check with your physician. Under certain circumstances, a nose, cough, and asthma medicine may contain one similar drug which could cause overdosage. Sometimes two entirely unrelated drugs can cause an unusual effect within someone's body.

A question often arises concerning when to take several prescribed drugs. Most drugs can be taken at exactly the same time. It is easier if someone is taking four drugs, to take them together whenever possible, so that one of them is not forgotten. If one, however, seems to cause an upset stomach or if certain drugs are to be given after meals or before meals, then these medicines would have to be taken separately.

If several drugs have to be taken every few hours throughout a day, it is very helpful if a schedule is prepared and followed. It is too easy to become confused and forget.

What is a suppository?

This is a drug which is given rectally. This form of treatment is needed when persons have vomiting and asthma. Suppositories can be wrapped in aluminum foil or paper. The covering should be removed before insertion into the rectum and the suppository should be greased with some kind of lubricant (i.e. cold cream). Suppositories hurt if inserted without extra lubrication. Inexpensive rubber finger covers can be obtained at pharmacies to protect the finger which puts the drug into the rectum. A suppository causes a sensation that the bowels need to be moved. Particularly, children should lie very still for a few minutes after insertion of the suppository. The tendency is to rush immediately to expel the suppository as the bowels are moved. It should be pushed in as far as your finger allows and then flipped sideways. If the bowels move *shortly* after inserting a suppository, directions must be obtained from a physician before giving the next one.

One advantage of a suppository is that often it can be inserted into the rectum of a sleeping child without awakening him. When properly used, they don't hurt any more than having a temperature taken rectally.

In general it can be stated that liquid rectal medicine is superior to suppository rectal drugs. Liquid medicine would be absorbed faster.

What should you do if you vomit shortly after taking drugs?

If vomiting occurs shortly after taking one or more drugs, check with your physician concerning when the next dose should be taken. If you vomit immediately, it may be possible to repeat the drug immediately. If the vomiting occurred, however, several minutes later, it could be dangerous to repeat the dosage. You might need your physician's help to determine why you are vomiting, and which drug might control this problem so that you would be able to take the medications necessary to control your allergies. (See page 209).

Are there many individuals who cannot take aspirin?

Aspirin can be a problem drug. It may dissolve on the tongue before it can be swallowed causing a bad taste. Less expensive forms of aspirin may dissolve less quickly than more expensive brands.

While most children are not allergic to aspirin, adults commonly have this problem. (See page 210). It is often difficult to detect aspirin allergy. For example, patients who have infection will frequently wheeze. Because of the infection, aspirin is taken. Later when wheezing is noted, it is assumed that it is related to the infection. The wheezing could be due to an aspirin sensitivity. (See page 26).

When should treatment be taken in relation to meals?

If a medicine is best absorbed or most beneficial when taken before, after, or between meals, it will be so specified on your prescription. If it is not specified, it indicates foods are unrelated to the effectiveness of that particular medicine.

Is the charge for a drug the same in all chemists?

Chemists may charge vastly different prices. To a degree, this will depend upon the size and owner of the drugstore.

If you buy a drug by its chemical name, it is much less expensive than if you buy a specific brand. For example, penicillin or acetyl salicyclic acid (aspirin) would be less expensive than if you purchased a particular type or brand of these drugs.

At what age should youngsters change from liquid to tablet drugs?

This depends upon the youngster. Some children prefer the pleasant taste of liquids in spite of a frequent disagreeable after-taste. Many children, over about 7 years of age, prefer to try to swallow a tablet or a chewable form of a medicine. Capsules have no taste, and are best for persons disliking flavoured medicines or drugs.

If an individual cannot take a pill, it is sometimes helpful if a bad-tasting liquid medicine is placed in a sweet heavy prune or grape juice. This helps to mask the flavour of the medicine. Pills can sometimes be crushed and placed in jelly, apple sauce, or a marshmallow.

Can a child be taught to swallow a pill?

Most children after the age of 7 years can learn to take tablet forms of medicine. Explain that tablets have less taste than liquid medicines. Practice using pill-sized sweet substances. Place the sweet "pill" far back in the centre of the tongue. Have the child drink a large swallow of water and try to wash the pill over the back edge of the tongue. When a youngster can swallow sweets in this manner, try half of a drug tablet.

How can a capsule be taken if it can't be swallowed?

The capsule contents can be placed in some nice tasting food such as jam, a marshmallow, pudding, ice cream, or creamy sweet. The contents should not be placed in a food to which someone is sensitive.

When should allergy medicines be discarded?

It is prudent to have allergy medicines available at all times even though you may not have had an asthma or hay fever attack for months or years. Sudden attacks may recur under unusual or inconvenient circumstances, when chemists are closed or physicians are not available. Always have emergency medicines available on holidays when you are away from home because new exposures could cause sudden symptoms. Most tablets or clear liquid medicines retain their potency for long periods of time but check with your pharmacist or physician. Don't use a tablet or liquid which has changed colour or take liquids which have precipitated or have particles floating in them. Throw away all old unlabelled medicines or drugs.

Is it safe to use drugs which have not been prescribed?

Persons with allergies should be cautious to use drugs prescribed for them alone. It is most unwise to use a friend's or relative's drugs or to allow a druggist to prescribe for you. This is the function of a physician.

Patients who have allergies should constantly remember that the ideal solution to an allergic problem is to eliminate what is causing the difficulty if this is possible. Drugs are helpful but it would be best if no treatment were needed.

Do vitamins help allergies?

There is no accepted scientific research at the present time that vitamins are beneficial for the treatment of allergies. There are some unsubstantiated claims that massive doses of vitamin C, B, and pantothenic acid are effective. Until their benefit and their safety have been confirmed, they cannot be recommended. Allergic children should maintain their usual vitamin supplements, especially if their diet is not adequate or well-balanced.

ANTIHISTAMINES

What is an antihistamine?

Drugs which relieve nose, eye, ear, and skin allergies are called antihistamines. These drugs may help stop the itching associated with hives and eczema. They also frequently decrease the itch of mosquito bites or insect bites.

Antihistamines decrease tissue swelling and reduce the production of mucus. Antihistamines are therefore helpful when a patient has stuffiness caused by nose tissue swelling or a runny nose caused by excessive mucus, as well as an itchy nose.

Are antihistamines always helpful?

No, some types of antihistamines do not help some people. There are different chemical categories of antihistamines. It is possible for one type to help an individual, whereas another type would be of no benefit at all.

When a patient has very severe hay fever or eczema, sometimes no antihistamines seem helpful. After that patient has started to respond to treatment, these same antihistamines may help to relieve symptoms.

What types of antihistamines are there?

There are liquid and tablet forms which last 4 to 12 hours, depending upon the brand. There are chewable or regular tablets which must be swallowed. Rectal or suppository forms of antihistamines are not available.

Antihistamines are also available as nose drops and sprays, and as eye drops. They can also be given by injection in an acute allergic emergency.

What is bad about antihistamines?

The most frequent bad effect from antihistamines is drowsiness or sleepiness. If the drug, however, relieves the allergy, use it at bedtime. Sometimes half the recommended dosage of a drug will relieve the symptoms and not cause sleepiness. If a drug is not helpful or sleepiness is a major problem, try a different antihistamine. Sometimes when an antihistamine is first taken, it causes sleepiness but this stops after a few days.

It is possible for antihistamines to cause your mouth to feel too dry or to cause abdominal discomfort.

A common side effect of antihistamines is a change in an individual's coordination. Adults should be careful when they drive cars if they are taking antihistamines and these drugs should be avoided prior to sports activities. In relation to this, exercise generally clears the nose, and so antihistamines might not be needed when someone is active. Once exertion is discontinued, however, nose symptoms often recur and then drugs might be needed again.

Adults must not drink alcoholic beverages when they use antihistamines, because this can cause extreme drowsiness. Antihistamines rarely cause blurred vision, difficulty in starting or stopping urination, low blood pressure (dizziness) or a fast heart beat. Antihistamines should not be used in creams or ointment forms applied to the skin because this might cause an allergy to develop to the antihistamine.

Do antihistamines vary in effectiveness?

An antihistamine might help a patient's mild symptoms but that same antihistamine might not be effective for severe symptoms. It is also possible for an antihistamine to be helpful over a period of several months and then gradually lose its effectiveness. At that point, a different antihistamine should be tried. It may be possible, months later, to return to the original antihistamine and find that it is again effective.

Do children and adults react similarly to antihistamines?

No, children and adults may respond quite differently to the same antihistamine. A child's dose of an antihistamine may make an adult very sleepy, while the adult dose may eliminate a child's symptoms and cause no drowsiness. There is a marked individual variation concerning tolerance to antihistamines, and it is difficult to predict how anyone will respond to any particular drug.

What symptoms indicate an overdose of antihistamines?

Initially, a patient could become extremely drowsy if a large overdose of antihistamine is taken. The drowsiness, however, is subsequently replaced by excitement and restlessness.

If a child or adult by mistake takes an excessive amount of antihistamines, an attempt should be made to cause vomiting by putting a finger down the throat. A physician should be contacted or the nearest hospital should be called. Strong coffee or caffeine is helpful to stimulate a person who is drowsy from antihistamines, but should never be used if the patient seems to be unduly excited.

Can an antihistamine help asthma?

In theory, antihistamines should help asthma and sometimes they do. They are not recommended, however, because they tend to dry mucus and this could be most undesirable in asthma. If lung mucus becomes thick and dry, it is more difficult to eliminate and this causes prolonged breathing difficulty. Antihistamines can safely be used with asthma drugs if patients have both nose and chest allergies. They should, however, not be taken if a patient has a *severe* asthma attack.

Do nose drops or sprays help?

Nose drops or sprays are sometimes beneficial in relieving both nose and ear allergies. Antihistamines may also help these same symptoms. Many physicians object to the use of nose drops because the tendency is to use them excessively causing nasal blockage called rhinitis medicamentosa. Nose drops or sprays should be used only as recommended by your physician (See page 25) and only for severe nose problems. For example, if a patient had taken an antihistamine but found sleep was impossible because his nose was stuffy, nose drops might temporarily relieve the problem.

How should nose drops be used?

Nose drops should never be used more often than 3 times a day for 3 days *unless* your physician specifies to the contrary. For exact details concerning how to use them, refer to page 25. The drops should be discontinued for 2 or 3 days after use for 3 days, and then can be used again for another 3-day period. By doing this, irritation of the inside of the nose can be prevented. If the nose is unbearably stuffy, one can use nose drops 3 times a day for 3 days on one side, and for the next 3 days, use drops on the other side. By alternating sides, there is always a breathing passageway and nose irritation from excessive nose drop use can be prevented.

Nose drops are available in different strengths for infants, children, and adults. For night use, there are long-acting nose drops. Parents must be careful not to use adult nose drops in children or infants, because certain types are much too strong.

ASTHMA MEDICINES

What forms of drugs are available for asthma treatment?
Asthma drugs are available in liquid, tablet, and capsule form to be taken by mouth, and in rectal liquid and suppository forms. Spray powders and liquids which are inhaled are also available. The dosage of drugs varies greatly according to weight and age. Asthma drugs which contain theophylline, must be taken carefully to insure that the correct dosage is not exceeded.

How do asthma drugs help?
They make it easier to breathe. They relax spasm of the air tubes and allow the airways to enlarge. They also help thin mucus so that it is easier to cough up. They diminish swelling of the lining of the air tubes, and this increases the efficiency of breathing.

What is Adrenaline?
This injected medicine helps immediately to relieve severe asthma. Most wheezing patients will breathe more easily within a few seconds or minutes. The usual form of Adrenaline is effective only for about 20 minutes, but longer acting forms are now available in some countries which can help up to 8 to 12 hours.
Adrenaline in any form will make the heart beat faster, but this is usually not any more harmful than exercising. This drug normally can make a person pale and nervous for a short period of time after it has been received.

What is ephedrine?
This is a form of medicine which is similar to adrenaline except that it is swallowed, not injected, to relieve asthma. It helps in about twenty minutes and the benefit continues for four to six hours. It can cause excitement or a jittery feeling but this is much less evident than it would be if someone received Adrenaline. If it causes a patient to feel uncomfortable, the drug should be discontinued or the dosage reduced.
There are several new forms of ephedrine available. These seem likely to replace ephedrine entirely in a few years' time because of their superiority. They open the air tubes more effectively while causing little stimulation of the heart. Some of these drugs, however, can cause a fine tremor of the hands.
In the past, ephedrine was frequently combined with a sedative or a tranquilizer because it caused excitation and a rapid pulse or nervousness in patients. There is presently a definite trend for physicians to recommend ephedrine alone rather than a combination of ephedrine plus some other drug.

Ephedrine may cause difficulty sleeping. Adults or children have also sometimes complained of difficulty either starting or stopping the flow or urine when they empty their bladder. This side effect is particularly liable to occur in men over sixty years of age.

What is theophylline?
Theophylline is available for patients in an oral, liquid, and tablet form and also as a rectal liquid or suppository drug. The oral liquid frequently has a most unpleasant taste, and some contain alcohol. If too much theophylline is taken it causes extreme nausea and vomiting of a coffee-ground-like material, headache, extreme restlessness, and agitation. If this type of problem is noted, contact your physician.

During severe asthmatic episodes, this drug is often given intravenously, but you *must inform* your doctor if you have taken any theophylline within the previous 8 to 12 hours because this could alter the intravenous dose which would be safe to use.

Recent studies have shown that theophylline is effective for different periods of time in different people. For this reason, your physician may have to individualize the dose of this drug to find out exactly how much you need and how often you need it.

Are mouth-spray aerosols helpful for asthmatics?
Young children cannot use aerosols because it takes a degree of coordination and cooperation which they do not possess. For the spray to be effective, the lips must be tightly around the mouthpiece. The patient must breathe through his nose. As the air is passing into the lungs, the aerosol is released into the mouth so it can also pass into the lungs. Each breath must be held as long as possible so that the drug has time to help when it is within the lungs. If there is a cloud of white coming from the mouth after using the spray, it indicates the medicine did not reach the lungs.

The major advantage of using a mouth-spray aerosol is that it helps in seconds. Some aerosols may help for a few hours, but most help less than one-half hour.

What are the disadvantages of pressurized atomizers (aerosols)?
There are many reasons not to use mouth-spray aerosols for asthma. The first is the strong tendency among older children and adults to over use spray medicine. They should never be used more than 3 or 4 times a day. If they are over used, they are seldom helpful. Overuse causes irritation of the throat, abdominal discomfort, and headache. Sprays tend to be habit forming.

There are excellent scientific studies which prove that some patients may seem to be better shortly after using asthma sprays, but subsequently their lungs go into severe spasm. Asthma can become much worse because sprays have been used. Sprays should be recommended only by your physician and never as routine treatment for asthma.

Are asthma and cough medicines similar?

They certainly may be. Cough medicines are of varied types and most combine one or more of the following ingredients in the mixture: ingredients to make mucus more thin, to decrease mucus production, to suppress the urge to cough, and to shrink swollen tissue. Asthma medicines often contain some of these ingredients. Cough and asthma medicine could, therefore, contain drugs which have similar actions. Check with your physician if you are using these two medicines at the same time.

Should narcotics be given to patients who have asthma?

Morphine and codeine are two commonly used drugs in medicine. Codeine is found in many cough preparations and is desirable to help relieve an irritating, dry, recurrent nightly cough often associated with infection. Narcotic-like drugs, however, are *not* desirable for asthma patients because they can interfere with normal breathing and sometimes aggravate asthma or coughing.

What is disodium cromoglycate?

The trade name in Great Britain and Europe is Intal made by Fisons Pharmaceuticals in various countries. In Canada it is sold also under the name of Aarane (Syntex Laboratories). Also sold as Lomudal.

How is it administered?

The drug, Intal, is a powder. It has to be inhaled through the mouth into the lung using a special inhalor called a spinhalor. A capsule containing the powder is placed in a capsule holder in the spinhalor. The capsule is pierced by moving a special part of the spinhalor up and down. The powder is taken into the lungs by breathing in a manner similar to smoking a cigarette. Each deep breath is held a few seconds before breathing out. It may take several breaths to empty the capsule of powder. Children over the age of 5 years can be taught to use it.

How many capsules should be used each day?

The amount of Intal needed, depends upon why it was being taken. If someone who has asthma near cats wants to visit a friend who has a cat, he may take a capsule before the visit. If the visit lasts over three hours or asthma symptoms occur, another capsule might be necessary after three hours.

Many patients require three or four capsules a day routinely to prevent wheezing. Patients will learn from experience how many capsules of

Intal powder they require. Some with pollen asthma will increase from one capsule to three or four as the pollen count (page 260) increases and slowly reduce the amount after three or four weeks. A school child may need more on days when he has strenuous exercise.

When does disodium cromoglycate (Intal) help?
The drug, which has virtually no known bad effects, is particularly useful in allergic asthma. It must be stressed that it *prevents* asthma but will not help when used during a wheezing episode. It is of particular value for children and adults who like to engage in strenuous sports exercise but find that their asthma does not allow them to do so. Intal prevents symptoms if used *prior* to a contact with allergenic items such as dust, pets, or foods. Patients of any age who have to take daily cortisone drugs may find that disodium cromoglycate helps so much that they may be able to stop using cortisone. This is particularly true of children.

When is disodium cromoglycate not helpful?
The drug is not helpful for those who are too young, sick, or too weak to inhale the drug or for some patients over the age of 60 years. It is not helpful for the patient who has emphysema or chronic bronchitis. Many patients who have intrinsic asthma are not helped, but a few are.

Does disodium cromoglycate help allergies other than asthma?
It can also be used for treating allergic nose problems. There is a special "insufflator" or nose inhaler which allows the powder to be puffed into the nose. The drug only *prevents* allergic reactions. It must not be used to treat a blocked or runny nose or to stop an episode of sneezing.
The drug has no use in any allergic skin condition, but has proven very helpful in some forms of eye allergy.

Can disodium cromoglycate (Intal) be used with other drugs?
Yes. All other asthma drugs can be used at the same time as disodium cromoglycate. When a patient first starts using Intal and finds it beneficial, it will be obvious that other asthma drugs can be taken in reduced doses or stopped because they are no longer needed.

Are there any other new medicines to help asthma?
Yes, there is a new form of powdered cortisone, which like disodium cromoglycate, is breathed into the lungs. A pressurized atomizer is used and the powdered drug goes directly into the lungs when the patient breathes in. It can easily be used by adults or most children over the age of five years. Cortisone taken in this form does not seem to cause any bad effects.

TREATMENT USED FOR SKIN ALLERGIES

What relieves itchy skin?
Calamine often decreases an itchy skin sensation. It might help relieve hives, eczema, mosquito or insect bites, or the areas which itch after allergy skin tests or extract treatments.

If menthol or phenol is combined with calamine, it sometimes increases the anti-itch effect.

Antihistamine drugs tend to decrease the urge to itch, but this may be partly due to the fact that these drugs often cause drowsiness. Antihistamines should not be used directly on the skin, because this might cause an allergy to develop to that particular antihistamine. Some skin preparations contain tars which diminish the urge to itch.

How helpful is cortisone skin medication?
Cortisone can be prescribed as a cream, ointment, lotion, or oil to help decrease redness and itching of the skin. Usually these are applied sparingly 4 or 5 times a day. A tiny speck should be placed every ½ inch or so over the itchy skin and these small specks should be rubbed or blended together using the tip of the finger. A thin layer applied often is far superior to one thick application each day. The skin rash may gradually improve, but *will recur* again unless the cause of the rash is determined and eliminated. Each time the rash recurs, cortisone may be needed again.

Is dry skin helped by the use of bath oils?
There is some disagreement concerning this, but there is no doubt that oil added to bath water causes the tub to become dangerously slippery. Oils which are left on the skin after an oily bath are more apt to be absorbed by the bath towel than the skin. For this reason, it is more beneficial to apply oil after bathing and drying the skin. The fundamental problem, of course, is not outside the skin, but inside; and an oil put onto the skin will help only temporarily.

An emulsifying ointment can be used as soap on the skin of patients who have eczema. The same ointment diluted with hot water to 8 or 10 times its original volume can be poured into the bath water.

CORTISONE (STEROID) MEDICINES

What is the function of cortisone or a steroid?
This is a hormone drug which is sometimes used to treat allergies and other medical problems. It is a powerful and essential drug which sometimes may be life saving. Like many similar powerful drugs, it has great

potential to help or to harm. This hormone is so potent that its use must always be closely supervised by your physician. Its major function is to decrease inflammation or swelling and redness which can occur in various areas or organs of the body for many different reasons. Although cortisone will relieve many medical problems temporarily, it does not cure allergy. It merely helps a patient through a critical period.

When would a physician prescribe cortisone?
It is used mainly when ordinary drugs do not relieve allergies. When a youngster cannot play normally and attend school, or when an adult cannot work or sleep, cortisone might be necessary. Life-threatening distressing emergencies (see page 110) can arise and this drug is sometimes effective in helping these allergic problems.

Is there a difference among cortisone preparations?
Yes. There is a marked variation in the potency and strength of cortisone preparations taken either by mouth or applied to the skin. The more powerful or beneficial a form of cortisone may be, the more likely that that particular preparation might have some undesirable effects. Your physician can decide which preparation is best and how long treatment should be continued.

Is cortisone dangerous if taken for short periods of time?
Patients may receive very large doses of cortisone during a critical emergency. The drug is generally discontinued within a few days as soon as the emergency situation is under control. Under these circumstances, there is relatively little danger and the drug is most worthwhile. (See page 113).

When could stopping cortisone be a problem?
If cortisone is taken by a patient for many weeks or months, it may be extremely difficult to stop the drug even though the dosage is gradually lowered. Patients who have eczema or asthma may find that whenever the dosage is lowered below a certain critical level, the symptoms become much worse. It can become a major challenge for a physician to stop this beneficial but potentially harmful drug. For this reason, many physicians are most reluctant to treat with cortisone. Cortisone preparations which are swallowed should *never* be stopped suddenly unless your physician has specifically advised that this be done. If this drug has been taken for weeks or months, it may be essential that the dosage be decreased slowly and gradually.

How dangerous is cortisone when it is used on the skin?
It causes relatively few undesirable effects, and is beneficial or helpful

when properly used to relieve certain skin problems such as eczema. Cortisone ointments or creams are frequently applied in relatively low concentrations to small areas of the body so that the effect is mainly local. If a strong concentration of cortisone is applied to large areas of the body, it is possible to absorb so much cortisone that some undesirable effects can be noted. (See page 62).

What undesirable minor effects does cortisone cause?

The common unpleasant minor effects from cortisone are: increased hairiness of the body or face, a rounding of the face, and a hump-like swelling on the back of the neck. Acne sometimes flares. There may be an increase in appetite and weight. Some patients have abdominal pain and bloating, a rise in blood pressure, or an itchy breast or rectal area. The urine may temporarily show an excessive amount of sugar. Patients may have difficulty sleeping. Adults in particular can have softening of their bones which may lead to a proneness to fractures. Children can have a mild to marked decreased growth in height. Other problems noted at times are excess perspiration, a dry mouth, fatigue, a flushed face, leg cramps, and easy bruising. Women may have menstrual difficulties.

What serious problems are sometimes noted after receiving cortisone?

Cortisone may cause an individual to feel fine when he isn't. For example, it can at times conceal the effects of infection so that you don't know you are ill. The combination of feeling well while an infection is spreading can be extremely dangerous. This is one reason that a patient who is receiving cortisone must be *examined* by his physician frequently "regardless" of how well he may feel. If a patient receiving cortisone feels unwell for any reason, or if he develops a fever or an obvious infection, his physician must be notified. A patient on cortisone may have pneumonia and a normal temperature. Most individuals who are *not* taking cortisone would feel unwell, and have a fever with a severe infection such as pneumonia.

How can cortisone's effect on growth be diminished?

If cortisone is used only for a few days, regardless of the dosage, it will not alter a child's height. If, however, this drug is given each day for prolonged periods of time in moderately high doses, it definitely can cause the growth in height to be less than normal. This effect is not noticed if cortisone is given every other day rather than every day.

This growth effect will be stopped if the daily use of cortisone can be stopped. When this hormone is discontinued, a sudden fast compensatory growth spurt in height often takes place which should allow a child to attain his predicted height providing he is still young enough to grow in height.

Some children unfortunately are so incapacitated by asthma that the physician has to make an extremely difficult decision. In spite of the fact that this drug is interfering with a child's growth and all the other problems this drug may cause, it may be essential that a child receive this medicine so that he can live a more normal life.

In Great Britain, newer forms of inhaled cortisone are available. Such small amounts of the drug are used that no side effect such as growth interference is noted. It is possible for most children and many adults to stop cortisone pills with the use of these newer preparations.

Should asthmatic children on cortisone be treated specially when immunized for measles?

Experience has shown that during a measles epidemic, hospitalized children on cortisone have measles similar to other children not on the hormone. The allergic asthmatic child, however, may have bad asthma for one or two months after receiving the measles vaccine.

Should a patient receive cortisone for many years?

Although it is not desirable, it may be essential for severely ill children or adults to receive this drug for many years. If this is necessary, patients should be aware of the minor and major undesirable effects of this drug, so their physician can be notified when problems arise.

After stopping cortisone, must it ever be restarted?

It is sometimes essential that cortisone be given again when it has not been needed for several months. A common reason to restart this drug would be a severe allergic reaction such as asthma. If someone needs certain types of cortisone for any medical reason over a long period of time, it can cause the adrenal glands, which are located above the kidneys, to shrink. These glands normally make cortisone, but if this hormone is received by a patient, either swallowed or by injection, the adrenal glands do not have to make as much cortisone as normal. It is similar to a factory that is making a certain product for which there is no longer a demand. The factory reduces production of that particular item. If there is a sudden great demand later on, the factory may not be able to make it quickly enough to satisfy the need. This problem arises in the human body during stress. When someone has a severe infection, has surgery, or if there is a family crisis, the adrenal glands have to produce more cortisone than usual. At that particular time, extra hormone is needed by the body to cope with the emergency situation. If the adrenal glands are not able to function adequately and supply enough cortisone when it is needed, your physician must give you an adequate amount. This may be true if a person has received cortisone within 6 to 12 months prior to a severe emotional or medical crisis. Check with your physician so that he can decide if more cortisone is necessary, and advise you accordingly.

ANTIBIOTICS

Are there different types of antibiotics?
There are two major categories of antibiotics. The first helps defend against gram-positive bacteria, and the second helps relieve infections caused by gram-negative bacteria. Common gram-positive bacteria include streptococcus which can cause sore throats, or pneumococcus which can cause pneumonia. There are, of course, many other types of germs which cause infections in these and other areas. Other infections are caused by viruses and we have no antibiotics which effectively help these.

When an infection is not better after a few days on an antibiotic, it could indicate that the wrong type may have been used or that it was a viral infection. The only way a physician can be certain concerning which antibiotic is best would be to culture the infected area. This means that some of the germs are removed from the infected area and grown on special germ food (cultured). The organisms are identified and special tests tell which antibiotic is best to eliminate the infection. Cultures of infected areas, however, often require days before the exact offending germ can be determined. For this reason, cultures are taken mainly in patients who have infections which are persistent and difficult to treat.

By examining the blood it is sometimes possible to tell the difference between a bacterial or viral infection.

If a patient takes an antibiotic, when will he start to improve?
Improvement may be noticed in several hours, but in general it requires a day or two before an individual is definitely better. If there is no improvement after 2 or 3 days, check with your physician.

Can an antibiotic help if a patient is not examined by a physician?
Yes, in general there would be no problem but sometimes difficulty could arise. For example, if someone is wheezing and has pneumonia, he may have been advised immediately to take an asthma drug and an antibiotic. If the patient, however, was not examined, it is possible that the antibiotic would be taken for only a few days and pneumonia could be partially rather than completely treated. Under such circumstances chest symptoms such as coughing could conceivably linger for an extended period of time. Partially treated pneumonia would be very difficult to diagnose if the patient had not been examined when the problem first began. For this reason, it is important for a physician to prescribe an

antibiotic only after the exact cause and location of the infection has
been determined.

How harmful or helpful is one or two days of an antibiotic?

Many individuals use a small supply of antibiotic left from a previous
prescription when they begin to have a new infection. This tendency can
cause major problems unless the patient is examined and the correct
antibiotic prescribed for *an adequate period of time.* For example, let us
suppose that the antibiotic which the patient took was the correct one to
stop the growth or kill the bacteria which were causing the problem.
During the first day or two the germs which are most sensitive to this
antibiotic are most apt to be killed or affected. If the antibiotic, however,
is stopped after 2 or 3 days only the strongest bacteria would have sur-
vived. These stubborn bacteria can begin to multiply and within a few
days infection again recurs. This time, however, the germs causing the
infection are resistant to the original antibiotic and the infection may be
more difficult to treat. For this reason, 1 or 2 days of an antibiotic not
only may not help an individual but actually may cause an infection to
become more difficult to treat.

CHAPTER TEN

A) Skin testing
B) Allergy injection treatment

What is a skin test?

An allergy skin test is one method of detecting or confirming the cause of allergy. The physician decides which substances are most probably causing a patient's allergy from his medical history. The more precise information an allergist has concerning when symptoms occur and what might cause the problem, the more selective the physician can be when he does testing. Possible allergenic suspects are placed on or just under the skin and this is called a skin test.

Why are skin tests performed?

There are a number of reasons to do tests for allergy. The history may not be accurate or known; so skin tests help detect unknown causes of allergy. The skin tests may help to confirm suspected allergies. Skin tests also help determine how sensitive a patient is to an item. Once testing is completed, an allergy extract is prepared which contains substances for which the patient needs treatment. If the skin tests indicated a strong allergy, the early extract treatments would have to be diluted or weakened. If the skin tests, however, revealed a slight or weak allergy, the beginning extract treatments could be given safely with stronger solutions of the allergenic substances.

How are skin tests done? How are they interpreted?

In general, there are two major types of allergy skin tests. There are scratch or prick tests done *on* the skin and intradermal tests which are done *in* the skin. Some physicians do only scratch tests, others do only intradermal and still others use a combination of both testing methods.

Scratch or Prick Tests

These detect strong allergies. By using this method it is possible to diagnose an allergy or to decrease the number of intradermal (needle) tests necessary to help determine causes of allergy.

Scratch tests are made by pricking the skin with a needle or a tiny pointed instrument. This technique causes little discomfort and seldom causes any bleeding. The skin is slightly indented or pricked, not cut. Testing can be done on the arms, thighs or back. A drop of the allergenic solution such as dust is placed on the skin before or after the area has been pricked. The solution maybe blotted or rubbed into the area of the prick. In about twenty minutes the skin test area is examined and the results interpreted. If the test site becomes red and itchy and looks a mosquito bite, this is a positive reaction and indicates that the patient is probably allergic to the substance tested. Positive reactions tend to disappear completely in about thirty minutes. If the skin test site appears unchanged after twenty minutes, this is a negative test. This means the patient is not allergic to the test substance, or that stronger tests of the intradermal type might be necessary to show the allergy.

Intradermal Tests

These tests are done by injecting a very tiny amount of an allergy solution into the layer of the skin. The tests are performed on the outer upper arms. The needle which is used is so tiny that little discomfort is noted by the patient. These tests can be interpreted in 10 minutes or so. Positive reactions cause mosquito-bite-like spots while negative reactions do not alter the skin test area. Tests for some allergenic items might first be done with a weak solution and if this causes no reaction, the tests might be repeated using a stronger concentration.

Persons who have strong allergies may have many positive reactions by the prick testing method or when the weaker intradermal skin test solutions are used. Persons with less allergy may show no reaction until strong intradermal tests are done.

Sometimes there is no immediate reaction at the skin test area but several hours later or the next day, the test site becomes red and itchy. This is called a delayed reaction. Your physician should be told when the reaction appeared, how large it became and how long it lasted.

Does skin testing cause allergic symptoms?

Sometimes mild allergic symptoms occur because of an extremely positive skin test reaction. Such reactions seldom occur.

How many skin tests are needed for allergic evaluation?

This varies markedly depending upon the patient's age and the severity and time of the year when symptoms appear. There are also personal preferences among individual physicians. In general, maybe 20 to 100 scratch skin tests or about 50 to 200 intradermal (needle under skin) tests might be done for a complete allergy study.

How many skin tests would be performed in one visit?

There is a marked variation depending upon the size and age of the patient and the allergist's method of testing. More tests would be carried out on larger children and adults, than on small patients. Twenty to thirty scratch tests can easily be performed on a small child without difficulty. The number of intradermal skin tests would vary from possibly 5 in a small child up to 40 or 50 in an adult.

Does a seasonal pollen allergy require many skin tests?

If a patient's symptoms occur each year at the same time for a very short period, only a small number of pollens or mould spores could be at fault. Testing would be necessary only for the few specific allergenic substances found in the air at that particular time.

Are skin tests painful?

Scratch or prick tests are not painful. On the back or lower arms they often tickle. An intradermal test feels like a slight pinch or prick in the skin.

Most children over 4 or 5 years of age can be tested without much difficulty. Children younger than 4, however, may be a challenge. Most children do not fear allergy tests and many look forward to their visits. Adults seldom complain.

Parents can convey fear or confidence to their youngsters. Some parents tell their child that the skin tests will be painful and hurt. This implants the idea that testing is going to be an uncomfortable experience. Other parents wisely give their child assurance without implying fear. A visit to the doctor should not be mentioned until time for the visit so nervous youngsters do not worry.

How reliable are allergy skin tests?

Most skin tests are reliable in that a positive reaction usually indicates allergy. Skin tests for pollens or inhaled substances are very reliable. A positive skin test, however, in itself is of little value unless it can be related to a patient's symptoms.

Some skin tests reflect past allergies. For example, if a patient were allergic to eggs as an infant and later "outgrew" this problem, the positive skin test for egg could remain. Most skin tests reflect present allergies which means that the patient has symptoms from the substance to which the skin reacted positively. Sometimes, a skin test may reveal a future allergy. A patient may have a strong reaction to grass pollen but no symptoms during the grass season. Within a couple of years such patients sometimes develop symptoms during the grass season.

Of all allergy skin tests performed, those for foods are least reliable because we cannot test for digested cooked foods and fresh fruits and vegetables are difficult to keep fresh for testing. It is possible to have a negative intradermal skin reaction to a food and be very allergic to the food. It is also possible to have a positive reaction to a food and to have no difficulty from that food. Scratch food allergy tests are more valuable and reliable than intradermal tests.

Some physicians believe that food testing carried out by placing drops under the tongue is more reliable. This is called a sublingual test. Many allergists strongly doubt the reliability of this type of test.

In the final analysis, the value of any food test is really in the eating. Regardless of the skin test reaction, the final answer rests with the patient. Can he eat the food without any difficulty?

Can a negative skin test reaction be incorrect?

This seldom happens. However, sometimes a patient is obviously allergic to grass. Although the symptoms recur each year during the pollen season, the grass skin tests are negative. If grass pollen is placed in the nose or eye, or breathed into the lungs, it is sometimes possible to prove an allergy to this substance. On rare occasions, a patient may have entirely negative reactions to all allergy testing methods, but respond well when treated for seasonal pollens.

Can a parent's skin be used for infant allergy tests?

It is possible indirectly to determine what is causing an infant's allergies by using a parent's skin but it is not as reliable as tests on the infant's skin. Tests do not cause so much discomfort that such an elaborate procedure is warranted under most circumstances. Infants seldom require many skin tests (See Chapter 7).

Do all patients who have allergies need skin tests?

No. At times it is possible from a patient's history to determine that a food, for example, might be the major or most likely cause of the patient's difficulty. In such an individual, dietary trials could be more rewarding than skin testing.

Other patients are sensitive to certain items and if their home is made relatively "allergy-free", as suggested in Chapter 11, the symptoms may subside.

If, however, home and diet changes do not relieve a patient's symptoms, skin testing would be necessary. A large percentage of patients seeing allergists require skin testing. Most patients who have significant symptoms during the warm months of the year when pollens and mould spores are a problem, need to be skin tested so that allergy extract therapy can be given.

Should certain drugs be avoided prior to skin testing?

Patients should not take antihistamines (to treat hay fever) or asthma drugs for at least 12 to 24 hours prior to allergy testing. Aspirin, antibiotics, disodium cromoglycate (Intal) and cortisone (steroids) do not significantly affect skin test reactions. Some cough medicines could alter skin reactions because they contain an antihistamine.

When should testing for a seasonal allergy be done?

Let us suppose that an individual has symptoms when grass happens to pollinate in the area where he lives.* Because it takes several months for allergy extract treatments to help a patient, it is necessary to have skin testing carried out 6 months prior to the time when symptoms start. If someone has grass allergy in June, allergy treatments should be started by January. This would allow adequate time for skin testing and for the patient to begin to receive benefit from allergy extract injection therapy.

Can skin testing be done if you're wheezing?

If the wheeze is severe, asthma treatment must be given. Notify your physician because testing cannot be performed at that time. Your physician might have to give you special asthma drugs to stop the wheeze.

If the wheeze is moderate or slight, check with your physician. Sometimes the testing can be scheduled when a dose of a drug is due. After allergy skin tests are completed, the usual drugs can be taken whenever necessary.

How often do skin tests have to be repeated?

Children from infancy to 5 years of age are prone to develop new allergies. Testing carried out during that period of time might have to be repeated in a few years. These children may develop different symptoms due to different allergenic substances as time passes.

Most adults have allergies which remain relatively constant and should improve on treatment. If, however, a patient who had been doing well developed symptoms at a time of the year when he previously seemed fine, testing for possible new exposures might be indicated. Many patients require occasional re-tests for items which could have been negative in the past. A dog skin test, for example, may be negative and sometime later become positive when a patient's symptoms become worse after acquiring a dog.

What does an allergist do after completion of skin testing?

Once the skin tests are completed and other laboratory studies have been carried out, an allergist will carefully evaluate the patient's history

*For pollen times see page 260.

and findings on physical examination. Recommendations are often made concerning the home and the diet. An extract of the allergenic substances to which the patient is sensitive may have to be prepared. All items which cause positive skin reactions cannot be placed in extracts, therefore, some recommendations are given concerning how to avoid these. For example, foods are not placed in extract medicines. A patient who has obvious food allergy should be informed concerning possible hidden forms of this food. (See page 168).

Some physicians prefer to give separate injections for each allergenic substance and others place several allergenic substances in a single extract so fewer injections are needed. Providing the patient improves, it does not matter which method is used.

What other types of tests do allergists perform?

A physician will determine which other tests are indicated depending upon the patient's symptoms, a chest X-ray and tests for tuberculosis or other types of infectious lung diseases might also be necessary. Special studies of breathing and lung function tests are sometimes done routinely on every visit to the doctor. If a patient has excessive lung mucus, some instruction concerning how to cough more effectively might be indicated.

If a patient had major nose or ear difficulties, sinus and adenoid X-rays might be helpful. X-rays to determine the size of adenoids, however, can be misleading.

Allergic persons often have an increased number of white blood cells, the eosinophils, in their blood. Excessive eosinophils also may be found in the nose, chest, eyes, ears or stool mucus. If these cells predominate, it often means that the patient has allergies.

Many young children and some allergic adults have an excessive number of infections. One portion of blood contains gamma globulin. This helps ward off infections. There are many other blood components which affect an individual's ability to fight infection. Special blood tests may show why some allergic patients have recurrent infections.

Substances which cause allergies are called antigens or allergens. Normally the body forms many types of antibodies against many types of antigens. Persons who have allergies often possess a special type of antibody called IgE or immunoglobulin E (skin-sensitizing antibody or reagin). It is this antibody which is responsible for positive skin test reactions. New methods of easily measuring IgE are being developed and in the near future it may be possible to examine a sample of a person's blood, instead of doing skin tests, to help determine what is causing someone's allergy.

It seems likely that eventually many different antibodies, other than IgE, which are directly related to some forms of allergy will be measured and studied from samples of blood. These tests may help greatly in the better detection of food or drug allergy.

TREATMENT WITH ALLERGY EXTRACTS

In this chapter the use of aqueous or "water" allergy-extract therapy will be discussed unless otherwise specified. In some countries allergy extract is called a vaccine.

There are many methods to give allergy-extract therapy. Although these methods may be dissimilar, it does not mean that they are ineffective.

Each physician individualizes his method of practice and although the answers are generalities, they reflect only our personal opinions based on our experience.

What is the theory behind allergy-extract treatments?

The basic premise is that a patient will develop gradual protection against the substances to which he is allergic if an extract of some of these substances is injected into this body. The dosage and strength of the extract solution is gradually increased so that the patient should form more and more protection.

Are allergy-extract injection treatments really helpful?

Some patients are helped only slightly and others improve dramatically. Adults respond almost as well and quickly as do children.

There is at present some controversy about why and how extract treatments help. It is embarrassing to allergists that they cannot explain to their complete satisfaction exactly why patients improve. This lack of knowledge, however, in no way alters the fact that patients who are receiving treatment usually have fewer symptoms.

When will allergy treatments begin to help a patient?

There is a marked variation among patients in relation to when they improve. Once allergy injections are started, a few patients notice they are using less medicine and having fewer allergies within 2 or 3 months. Many see obvious improvement in 6 to 8 months. Some do not improve at all or are not better for a year or two.

If a patient is responding well to therapy, he should notice that as time passes he has fewer allergic episodes and needs less medication. Each year should be better than the previous one.

Which allergenic substances are included in extracts?

Some allergists prefer to use extracts which contain a single or a few items. Other combine similar items such as several tree, weed and grass pollens into one extract. Still others combine many dissimilar allergenic substances into one extract. There are advantages and disadvantages to each method, but the most important consideration is whether a patient improves or not.

In general, extracts can contain dust, mites, feathers, cotton linters, kapok, mould spores and tree, grass and weed pollens. Bacterial vaccines are sometimes included although their effectiveness and use is controversial. Some allergists believe them to be extremely effective whereas others believe them to be of absolutely no value.

Which substances are *not* included in allergy-extracts?

Insecticides, cottonseed, flaxseed, silk, wool, cigarette smoke and foods are usually not incorporated into extract treatments. Animal danders may or may not be used. (See Chapter 13). In general, all of these substances can be avoided to varying degrees. Injections of extracts of these items are either not possible or they are not found routinely to be beneficial for patients.

Can allergy treatment be given for air pollution?

Extract therapy can be given for pollen and mould spores. Extract therapy, however, cannot be given for industrial waste, gaseous or chemical pollution.

How often should allergy extract injections be given?

When a patient first begins to receive extract therapy, his allergist will prepare a special individualized schedule. In general, a small amount of a weak solution is given and gradually the strength and dosage is increased to a level which is best for a patient or to an arbitrary top tolerated maximum level. The top dosage for one patient could be 1,000 times more than the dose needed by another patient to stay well. After a patient has received all his preliminary injections, he then needs to receive his maximum maintenance dosage repeated approximately every month.

Again there are many individual variations and some children or adults require their injection therapy as often as once a week to keep well, while others tolerate a 5 week interval without difficulty.

The frequency of treatments after a patient starts therapy is dependent upon several factors.

1. If a patient were very ill, treatments might be given as often as three times weekly on alternate days so that protection could form as soon as possible.

2. If a patient were very sensitive to allergenic substances and needed many (about 40) preliminary injections before his maximum dosage could be given, he might also need treatment several times weekly.

Treatments once a week would require 10 months, while injections three times a week would require only 3.5 months.

3. If a patient has seasonal symptoms requiring many treatments to attain his maximum extract level prior to the pollen season, he might need frequent injections. For example, if a patient needed 20 treatments to reach the top dosage and had 10 weeks before the pollen season started, he would need 2 treatments a week. If, however, there were 20 weeks before the next pollen season, he would need an injection treatment only once a week.

4. Some patients tolerate a 4 week schedule during the winter months, but might need treatments once or twice a week during the pollen season to stay well.

5. If a patient is not responding as well as desired, a physician often has two major choices in relation to extract therapy. If the allergy extract does not cause an excessive reaction in the area of the injection, the dosage can be increased. For example, a patient who receives 0.2 ml. (2 drops) without difficulty can gradually have his dosage increased. If, however, excessive swelling occurs from a dosage of 0.2 ml., the dosage cannot be increased further. Under such circumstances the maximum tolerated dose (0.2 ml.) can be repeated weekly or bimonthly in an effort to give that patient more protection.

What are the 3 most commonly used allergy-extract schedules?
The 3 schedules used to treat patients are classified as perennial or year-round, pre-seasonal, or co-seasonal.

The perennial schedule means that the patient's dosage is gradually raised to the maximum tolerated level. The patient continues to receive booster injection treatments *throughout the year* at about a monthly interval. This form of therapy is very effective. Patients require only about 12 injections each year.

Pre-seasonal therapy is recommeneded for some patients who have seasonal pollen problems. This form of treatment requires no injection treatments during the cold winter months. Instead treatments are needed 2 or 3 times a week for several weeks prior to the pollen season. This method is effective and beneficial for some patients, but can be inconvenient because of the need for frequent office visits.

Co-seasonal therapy refers to injection therapy given during a pollen season. When a patient is first seen by an allergist during a pollen season, treatment can be started and the injection treatments given at least twice a week. This form of treatment would be much less helpful than the other types of therapy. It, however, might be the only treatment possible for a particular individual. Many allergists do not use this method because it has not been found to be helpful.

It is possible for some patients to receive perennial treatment throughout the year. Because of a seasonal flare of their symptoms, they may need additonal co-seasonal treatment. This combined form of therapy is sometimes beneficial.

Is it important to receive injection treatments on time?

Allergists do not all recommend the same frequency for extract therapy. In general, it is not harmful to receive an extract on a date *earlier* than recommended by your physician. In other words, if you have to leave town or go on a holiday, it is certainly not harmful to receive your allergy-extract treatment a week or two earlier than normal.

If a patient is starting allergy-extract treatments, they may be received 2 or 3 times a week. If a patient misses one or several appointments, it is not usually critical. Missed treatments, however, would prolong the time needed before improvement would be noted.

When the dosage of a patient's extract is gradually being increased, treatments must be received at least every 14 days or the extract dosage cannot be raised. A patient's dosage can be increased only if he had no difficulty with the last injection treatment.

Most allergy patients eventually receive a satisfactory maintenance dosage every 4 or 5 weeks. If, however, a patient on a 5-week schedule, comes for his injection treatment on the 37th day, it might be unsafe for the physician to repeat the previous dosage. For safety reasons, the patient's dosage might have to be decreased. He might have to return after a short period of time so booster injections could be given to raise his extract dose to the previous top maintenance level. This causes the inconvenience of extra visits to the doctor.

Where should allergy extracts be injected?

No particular location seems to be best. It is a matter not only of the physician's but the patient's personal preference. All treatments, however, must be given so that a tourniquet can be applied *above* the site of the injection if an emergency arose. Some physicians prefer to give treatments in one arm on one month and in the opposite arm the next month. Occasionally, however, a patient will find treatments are painful when given into one arm but not the other. Some patients prefer treatments given either relatively high or low on the arm. If a patient finds that his injection treatment causes discomfort, he should discuss the problem with his physician. Changing the location of the injection may eliminate the problem.

What is a normal response to an extract treatment?

Normal responses include:
1. No visible reaction.
2. A tiny area of redness, itching or swelling not larger than about 3.5

cm. in diameter and not raised more than approximately 0.6 cm. The swelling should not last more than a day or two.

When patients first begin allergy-injection therapy, a small hive-like reaction is often noted. Although the extract gradually becomes stronger, the local reaction becomes less because the patient begins to form protection. When the patient is near his top-tolerated level a local reaction in the area of the injection treatment may reappear. It can become larger with each treatment but should not cause undue discomfort.

An allergy treatment should never cause excessive pain. If, however, someone accidentally bumps the area of the injection, for example while sleeping, it may hurt.

What is an abnormal *local* reaction to an allergy-injection?

An abnormal *local* reaction to an allergy-extract is one which causes excessive swelling or pain in the site of the treatment. Injections should not interfere with the patient's dressing, writing or eating. It is an abnormal reaction if the swelling extends from the elbow to the shoulder or if the arm is unduly painful, sore or itchy for a couple of days.

Are abnormal reactions to extracts ever *not* localized to the site of the injection?

The following list includes possible signs and symptoms of *generalized* reactions.

These can occur in any sequence or combination and vary markedly in severity. None of the following should occur, *even in a mild form*, during the 2 hour period after receiving an allergy extract. If symptoms are evident prior to a treatment which are *not* worse afterwards, the extract injection is not at fault. If symptoms suddenly appeared or if previous symptoms worsened significantly after treatment, it would indicate an abnormal response. This should be discussed with your physician, *before* the next treatment is given.

Nose
Stuffiness
Itching
Sneezing
Watery Discharge

Eyes
Redness
Itching
Watery Discharge

Mouth
Swelling of Lips or Tongue
Itching within Mouth
Throat Clearing
A Hoarse Voice

Skin
Small Welts or Nettle Rash
Generalized itching of the skin in an area other than the site of the
    injection
Itching in particular of the palms or the creases of the arms.

Chest
Shortness of Breath
Coughing
Wheezing

Miscellaneous
Headache
Abdominal Pains
Cramps
Diarrhoea or Vomiting
Red Earlobes
Uterine Contractions or Vaginal Bleeding
Irritability
Unusual Fatigue
Strong Heart Beat

What should a patient do for a reaction to an allergy extract?
A. If the reaction is a slight *local* reaction, confined to the site of the injection, the following might be helpful:
    1. If the area itches or seems red, give an antihistamine (See
page 103).
    2. If the area is swollen or hot, apply ice, not heat, and do not massage.
    3. If the area is painful give aspirin or an aspirin substitute (See
page 101). The dosage of aspirin for an adult 60, 120 or 300 mg. tablets.
For a child the dosage is a 60 mg. for each year of age up to the age of 5, so
that a 3-year-old would require 180 mg. every 4 hours. Aspirin tablets are
available in different strengths for children and adults.
    4. If the allergy injection site is painful, itchy and swollen, take an
antihistamine, an aspirin substitute and apply ice. A sling is helpful if the
arm is painful if it is not supported.
    If any of the above treatment is needed after an extract treatment, your
physician should be notified *before* the next dose of extract. Such infor-

mation could alter the dosage, time or method of giving the subsequent treatment.

B. For an abnormal reaction which affects some area of the body *other than* the site of the injection, the following should be done:

1. If you are still at the physician's, ask to see the doctor immediately so that you can be examined.

2. If you are en route home, pull your car to the side of the road and immediately take both an antihistamine *and* an asthma remedy. If going home in public transport, carry a small quantity of both of these drugs at all times so that they can be used for an emergency. If the reaction is severe, immediately return to your physician.

3. If you are home when the reaction occurs, you can promptly take your usual antihistamine *and* asthma treatment and immediately call the physician who administered the extract.

4. If the reaction to the injection treatment is alarming also apply ice to the area of the injection. A tourniquet may or may not be applied. If one is used it must be released at least once every 10 minutes.

Patients should not be alarmed that reactions are going to occur when they receive allergy-extract treatments. These problems *seldom* arise, but if they do, it is better for you to know exactly what to do.

Why would a severe abnormal reaction occur from a treatment?

There are many reasons why reactions occur in persons who never have had difficulty before. A common reason is probably because no one can see where an injection is being given. If it is injected near to a major blood vessel, the solution can be absorbed very quickly and it has the same effect as being exposed suddenly to a large amount of allergenic material.

Do severe abnormal allergic reactions occur very often?

Fortunately this type of reaction occurs very seldom because the dosage of extracts are usually increased very slowly and cautiously.

Is it possible to prevent a severe reaction to an allergy extract?

Yes, you can help prevent the occurrence of a severe reaction by remaining in the doctor's waiting room for at least 15 minutes after you receive your treatment. If you notice any sign or symptom of a slight reaction (See Page 127) immediately notify your doctor. He can give treatment and prevent the reaction from becoming severe.

If you notice that the *local* reaction to your allergy-extract treatment is gradually becoming greater with each subsequent treatment, it often indicates that you are near your top-tolerated dosage of extract. You should inform your physician about this *before* the next treatment is given, so that appropriate adjustments can be made.

It is not unusual for a physician to ask a patient if he had any difficulty from his last extract treatment and he casually says "no". After the injection treatment is given, he recalls that his arm was unusually swollen, or that he sneezed a few times after the treatment. This information should have been given to the physician or nurse *before* the injection treatment, not afterwards. By doing this you may be able to prevent a severe reaction from occurring. A large local reaction causes discomfort but is not really harmful.

What symptoms are *not* caused by allergy-extract therapy?

Extracts rarely cause a fever. If a fever is noted shortly after a treatment, it may indicate a coincidental infection and not a reaction to the extract. Allergic reactions to treatments usually occur within 2 hours after an injection. If symptoms appear more than 2 hours after a patient's treatment, it is possible but unlikely that it was caused by the extract. If a patient reacts to his treatment there is usually a local reaction at the injection site, as well as allergic symptoms elsewhere.

Rarely an individual receives an extract on one day and wheezes the next day. All patients are individuals, however, and some react in a manner different from most. If you *repeatedly* find that your extract treatments always cause a certain type of reaction, you should definitely discuss it with your allergist.

Are any mild symptoms often noted after extract treatments?

It is not unusual for children in particular to notice that they are tired, listless and not too hungry after they have received their treatment. This feeling of fatigue sometimes can be completely eliminated by decreasing the extract dosage by a small amount. This type of reaction is not serious.

What precautions should be taken when receiving allergy-extract treatments?

Always remain in your doctor's office for 15 or 20 minutes after receiving an allergy treatment. Wait even though treatments have been received for many years without difficulty. If the waiting room is too crowded, wait in your automobile or in the vicinity of the office. If a severe reaction occurs (See page 126) it is most apt to occur within 20 minutes. No one can help you as quickly or as well as the physician. Wait, even if you live near the doctor's office.

If you have a reaction to an allergy treatment, wait at least 1/2 hour after any future injections. Persons who react are more prone to have future reactions than patients who never have had difficulty.

A child receiving extract should always be accompanied by an adult. The parent should observe his child for approximately 2 hours after the treatment. It is during this period of time that reactions are most apt to occur. Avoid extract injections on days when sports activity or strenuous exercise is scheduled.

All patients should always carry an antihistamine and an asthma medicine (See page 106) in their car or in their purse so that if sudden allergic symptoms occur, *both* medicines can immediately be taken to relieve the problem. Liquid medicines are faster acting than tablets. An allergic reaction may begin with a sneeze or an itch, but within seconds or minutes asthma, coughing and body swelling can occur. This can happen in individuals who have never had welts or asthma. To be forewarned is to be forearmed.

If you have symptoms, how can you tell if you are reacting to an allergy injection?

If your nose was slightly stuffy or you were wheezing a bit before you received your extract treatment and you continued to have the same symptoms, you should not be concerned, If, however, the nose or chest symptoms suddenly become severe, this could indicate you were reacting. The area of the injection treatment may become more red and swollen than usual. If this is noted, follow the recommendations on page 127.

Are treatments needed more often than every 4 weeks?

Sometimes. Many patients notice no difference in their symptoms when they receive extract therapy every 4 weeks. Some adults and children, however, notice that allergic symptoms are more evident a few days before each monthly treatment. This could indicate that the injections are not being given at the optimum frequency. If symptoms occur 3 days before each monthly injection, the treatment should be given every 25, not 28 days.

After several months, the interval sometimes can be prolonged. If a patient does as well on a 4 week schedule as he does on a more frequent interval, he should be on a 4 week schedule.

Why should a patient suddenly need frequent allergy injections?

This is recommended when a patient needs an increase in his extract dosage to give him more protection, for example, prior to a pollen season. Sometimes patients need frequent "booster" treatments during a troublesome season. The interval between treatments can be prolonged again to the previous interval, as soon as the pollen season has passed. Not all patients are helped by such therapy.

Why does fresh, new extract necessitate extra treatments?

A single supply of extract lasts approximately 8 to 18 months. As the extract is being used, although it is refrigerated, it gradually becomes weaker. This means that new, fresh extract is stronger and the dose must be lowered and reraised again to the usual maximum.

Can a person's response to an extract change?

As time passes most patients become less sensitive to their extract and the reaction in the area of the injection becomes less evident. Once in a while the opposite occurs. A patient may notice an extremely strong reaction to a dose of extract which never caused difficulty previously. If this happens, your allergist will correct the problem.

Should a patient with an infection receive his extract?

There is a difference of opinion concerning this among physicians. Many allergists believe that if a patient has a slight infection the injection treatment can safely be given. In any particular patient, however, the physician in charge must make the final decision concerning whether treatment is to be given or not. If a patient has a high fever and feels most unwell, the infection should be treated. The allergy treatment should be delayed until he feels better.

Some children have infections and wheeze so often that it would be impossible to give an extract treatment if the chest had to be clear before the treatment were given. If a patient has an infection and is due for an allergy-extract treatment, the longer he waits for treatment, the greater the chance his asthma will become a major problem.

Should pregnant women receive allergy injection treatments?

Some allergists recommend that routine treatments not be given during the pregnant period. Others allow injection therapy but urge caution to avoid an allergic reaction (See page 126). Care must be used when raising or repeating an extract dose, especially during a pollen season. It should be stressed that pregnant patients should not be overdue or late for their allergy treatment.

Are sports activities permissible shortly after receiving an allergy extract treatment?

It would be best if at least 2 hours elapsed between an allergy injection of extract and a sports endeavour. Have the treatment given into the left arm, for example, if you plan to engage in some activity using your right arm. Take no antihistamine unless it is essential because this medication can interfere with normal co-ordination. Adults and older children should, however, always carry a chewable antihistamine and an asthma drug for emergency use.

Can a wheezing patient receive allergy injection treatment?

Yes. Many physicians give allergy-extract treatment although a patient is wheezing slightly. If wheezing were severe, however, it might be more essential to treat the patient's asthma. The examining physician would have to decide what was best.

How many years do patients need allergy injection treatments?

If a patient's symptoms are mild and have been evident only for a few months, he would require treatment for a shorter period than someone who had severe symptoms for many years. Children often respond more quickly to allergy-extract therapy than do adults.

Injection therapy should be given until no symptoms of allergy are noted from substances *for which a patient has received treatment* for a full two or three year period. Allergy-extract therapy is usually continued for several to many years. Severe symptoms might necessitate therapy throughout a patient's life-time so that a normal life is possible.

A patient possibly may be able to shorten the duration of allergy treatment by several years if detailed records are kept as suggested on pages 11 and 12. The more specific information which your physician can be given, the easier it is for him to decide when it is safe for treatments to be discontinued.

What happens if allergy treatment is stopped too soon?

Some individuals may be fortunate. Their symptoms may not recur or may remain mild. Many patients who discontinue treatments too soon, however, will remain well only several months before the original problems recur.

Adolescents are often most anxious to discontinue therapy. The final decision should rest with the physician and the patient's parents for their major concern will be solely what is best for the youngster's health.

Can a patient's symptoms recur after a physician's recommendation to stop therapy?

Yes, this can happen. While many patients remain entirely free of symptoms after stopping allergy treatments, a few will do poorly. Some have a recurrence of symptoms within a few months or years and therapy must be resumed. Most patients fortunately respond well and quickly once they are again receiving their allergy-extract treatments.

What should a patient do if allergy treatment is not helpful?

If a patient has shown no improvement after receiving allergy-extract treatments for 2 or more years, the entire problem should be discussed with your allergist. By thoroughly evaluating all aspects of a patient's allergies, changes often can be recommended which will provide greater relief. Some of these recommendations are suggested on page 133.

Why would a patient who did well on allergy extract therapy, suddenly do poorly?
Patients who have few or no symptoms for a long period of time sometimes find they are suddenly ill quite often. They may be helped if they honestly review the list of original suggestions and recommendations made by their allergist. A few common factors which should be considered are listed below.
1.   Has your home changed in any dramatic way? Is the bedroom, for example, less "allergy-free" than it was before? Is it dusty? Is it cluttered? (See Chapter 11).
2.   Has the bedroom been changed in location or have the contents of the room been altered? Has the mattress been changed? Are the mattress and box springs *entirely* encased in plastic? Are the encasings torn? Is the mattress cover wiped clean each week when the linens are changed? Is the bedroom heating outlet dusty? Was the bedroom carpet removed, covered or is it being vacuumed daily?
3.   Have you acquired any new sources of allergy such as a furry pet, carpet, stuffed furniture or different hobby?
4.   Have you moved to a new home and not discussed this with your allergist?
5.   Have you changed your heating system? Is the furnace filter being changed each month? Does your vacuum cleaner spill dust because the connections are not tight. Is your air-purifier working properly? Is the humidifier functioning well?
6.   Have you remodelled, painted or refurnished your home in any way.
7.   Has the basement been flooded or is your home more damp than usual? Is the dehumidifier functioning properly?
8.   Have you started to eat even a little bit of the food which you previously found to contribute to your symptoms? (See Chapter 12).
9.   Were the original dietary studies properly carried out exactly as your physician recommended? Was interpretation altered by an infection or some unforeseen happening? Were many mistakes made during the dietary trial which would make it difficult to interpret whether a food were a factor?
10.   Have you kept detailed records of possible factors which might be related to your allergic symptoms? (See page 11). Can you note any similarity or any item which seems repeatedly to be a possible factor?
11.   Have you noticed that the symptoms seem to be worse or better the week before or after allergy extract treatment. (See pages 130 to 132).
12.   Was your dosage of extract decreased when fresh allergy extract was obtained and never raised to the maximum level again? Have you repeatedly been overdue for your allergy extract treatment? (See page 123).

13.   Do you cough up a small amount of green or yellow mucus which could indicate a chronic low-grade infection in the sinuses or the lungs? If this is true, discuss it with your physician.

14.   Do your symptoms seem to occur the same time or day each week? Is there anything unusual about the period before you notice your difficulty. For example, some women are worse the day they do certain cleaning. A leaky vacuum cleaner could spew dust and cause symptoms for about 24 hours. Are you worse the day you do the laundry because the clothes dryer is not vented properly?

Can severe pollen symptoms be helped?

Sometimes, before or in spite of extract therapy, a patient may have severe symptoms during an unusually heavy pollen season.
The following might be helpful:

1.   An air purifier can be placed in the patient's bedroom during the pollen season to help reduce pollen exposure during the night hours. (See page 154).

2.   Different antihistamine, asthma or other drugs might be beneficial.

3.   The bedroom should be made as free of allergenic substances as possible. (See pages 139 to 145).

4.   The patient should remain indoors, if possible, and avoid rides in the country or activity which could cause excessive pollen exposure (cutting grass).

Can relatives or friends give a patient his allergy extract?

Some physicians might find this objectionable, while others do not. It is possible to cause a medical emergency by giving an allergy-extract treatment as explained on page 125. Reactions seldom occur but when they do, experience, medical knowledge and cool judgement are essential Medical equipment and techniques might be indicated which could be provided only by a physician.

If you are considering giving your child or yourself allergy-extract therapy consider how you would feel if some unforeseen and dangerous accident occurred. Safety, not convenience, should be your prime consideration.

Is it best to receive allergy-extract treatments from your regular physician or from your allergist?

An allergist who personally administers extract therapy is in a better position to provide regular supervision for all aspects of an individual's allergies.

Some countries, however, have only a few allergists. In such areas a local physician would administer the allergy extract therapy and aid the patient in following the suggestions and recommendations made by the allergy specialist. If problems or questions arose, consultation with the allergist would be advisable. In some countries it is not unusual for patients to give their own injections providing they have never had an untoward or abnormal reaction to the allergy extract.

Is it possible to mix two extracts in the same syringe?

In most patients it makes little difference if extracts of the same type are mixed together or given singly. Your physician can advise you.

What do bacterial vaccines contain?

A vaccine is composed of bacteria or germs known to cause infection. These bacteria have been killed so that they cause no disease when they are injected. This type of treatment is sometimes recommended for youngsters who have frequent asthma precipitated by injection. At times bacterial vaccines are combined with other allergenic substances into a single extract.

Are there different types of bacterial vaccines?

There are stock types of bacterial vaccines composed of common types of killed bacteria. Autogenous bacterial vaccines can be prepared from the specific germs found in an individual's lung mucus or nose secretions.

The effectiveness of both stock and autogenous bacterial vaccines is continually challenged. Many doctors do not feel that this form of treatment is helpful in any way. Other physicians, however, have the opposite impression.

What is alum precipitated extract treatment?

There is one form of *long-acting* allergy extract which uses alum to precipitate the allergenic substance prior to extract preparation. The suspended particles are injected into the patient allowing the allergenic substances to be absorbed more slowly.

What are the advantages of this form of treatment?

When a patient begins to start his allergy treatments, fewer injections than usual would be required with alum precipitated extracts before reaching a person's maximum level. Once the patient is receiving his maximum dosage, booster injections may be needed less often (every 6 weeks rather than 4). This type of treatment sometimes helps patients who cannot tolerate or have not responded well to the usual aqueous form of allergy extract therapy.

What are the disadvantages of this form of treatment?

One problem is that more frequent and severe reactions occur in the area of the injection causing swollen arms. This is true particularly for dark-skinned individuals. Reactions from an alum extract occur anytime from one half hour after treatment to the following day. Reactions can occur at inconvenient times when medical help is not readily available.

Is it harmful for an extract to be kept at room temperature?

A sterile extract can be exposed to room temperature for several days or weeks without significant alteration. This occurs whenever an extract, for example, is mailed to an individual who lives a great distance away from his allergist. Extracts should be kept refrigerated, but *not* frozen as much of the time as possible.

Is it possible to give allergy-extract treatments by mouth?

It is not believed that allergy-extract therapy can be given by mouth because the allergenic substance would be digested in the stomach and intestines. This could alter the protection which would develop. One school of allergists, however, treat patients by placing drops of allergenic substances under the tongue, and claim that this form of therapy is helpful. Investigations are being carried out at the present time to verify or deny the effectiveness of such therapy.

CHAPTER ELEVEN

Making a home allergy-free

How can you tell if your home is causing allergies?

If you find you are well whenever you are not in your home and shortly after you return home you are sick, it points to something within the home as the cause of your problem. You may find you are better when you are on a vacation; when you are in the hospital, or visiting friends. If you are somewhat worse during the colder months of the year when the house is closed and you spend an increased amount of time inside, it often means a home allergy. Such persons are often worse during the night or as soon as they arise in the morning.

If you are unsure, visit a friend, go camping, go to a hotel for a few days, even rent a trailer and see whether your problems disappear completely or not in the different environment. You must be careful when you do this, however. Do not take anything with you to your temporary home because the item which you carry could conceivably be the substance in your home causing difficulty. For example, you should not take your favourite pillow, your body powders, or your pet. Foods are not significantly related to your symptoms if you are always better when you are away from home and your diet has remained essentially the same.

Sometimes you can be fooled because the place you visit contains the same allergenic substances that you have in your home. For example, if you visit a dusty old home where there are pets you may not improve.

Is it important to make your home allergy-free?

It is sensible to make your home allergy-free if you have allergy symptoms either every day, or on and.off throughout the year. If, however, you have difficulty only during certain seasons of the year when pollens or mould spores are in the air (See page 260), home changes would not be as important. During the pollen season, an allergy-free bedroom might, however, help to reduce your symptoms. (See page 143).

Some patients initially have symptoms only during certain pollen seasons and subsequently notice allergy problems persisting throughout the year.

If allergy precautions are taken in a person's home, it helps prevent others in the home from developing allergy. Individuals who enthusiastically change their home so it is more allergy-free, are often rewarded by noticing that their symptoms decrease quickly. Many patients have excuses, valid and imaginary. If they cannot or will not make their home allergy-free, their allergies may persist.

Where should an allergy-free home be located?

Try to find a location which is away from trees, fields or factories. While rural areas have more pollen, urban areas have more air pollution.

Select a home which is not near heavily used roads, industrial areas or railroads, airports, stables, barns, petrol stations, dumps, mills, garages or parking sites. Some health departments can give information concerning air pollution in surrounding areas and weather stations can tell you the prevailing winds in your area. The wind, if possible, should blow *away* from your home so pollens and factory odours will not be blown towards the house.

Live in a home located in a relatively high area of land because low areas such as river bottoms are sometimes flooded and this can create mould spore contamination problems. In addition, mites (See page 142) in household dust are more prevalent in damp homes.

When purchasing a home, it is wise to check the basement to be certain there is no water-level mark which would indicate previous flooding. If the soil near the house is very shaded, grass frequently will not grow, and the home is more likely to be mouldy or damp.

Do not select a home in a locale which conducts large scale spraying with insecticides for mosquito or tree problems. If such a problem exists, take your vacation during the period of time when this is being done.

Is the age of a home important?

Extremely old homes can seldom be made allergy-free. Very new homes can cause irritation supposedly from plaster dust. Newer homes, however, are definitely preferable to very old ones. Purchasing a home, and subsequently remodelling it, often causes allergic symptoms because of excessive exposure to dust and irritation from paint and various solvents.

Regardless of the type of home in which one lives, be certain that it is not draughty. Seal windows with caulking material and use weather stripping around the doors. Cord caulking can easily be removed when the weather is warm. Replace it when the cold season begins.

If someone has pet allergies, do not purchase a home if the previous owner raised or kept animals in the house. This can cause persistent problems which last as long as that individual lives in that house.

If you live in an apartment, select one which is relatively new, but old enough that new construction odours are gone. Such odours include the smell of paint, plaster, tar or asphalt.

How can you tell which room is causing allergies?

The easiest way is pay close attention to the sudden occurrence of symptoms.

If the allergies are worse during the night or on arising, it may be due to something in the bedroom. If symptoms are worse after entering or leaving a bathroom, it might be related to some substance or odour in that area. If symptoms occur only in the kitchen, it could be caused by an odour or certain foods. A sudden coughing spell, tightness of the chest, or series of sneezes, should alert you to a recent exposure which caused the allergy symptoms. If, for example, a child is always sitting in a certain chair or playing with a specific toy when symptoms occur, be suspicious of everything in that particular area.

BEDROOM

Is the bedroom often a cause of allergy?

It is certainly is. This is the one room where people spend more time per day than in any other room. In a 24-hour period, children will spend 8 to 10 hours in their bedroom. An individual may be able to tolerate daytime exposure to things causing allergy without having major difficulties, but if he is also exposed all night, he may have symptoms because of excessive contact with allergenic substance.

It is impossible (and unnecessary) for a busy housewife to keep the entire home allergy-free. For this reason the bedroom is very important. If only one room is to be kept allergy-free, it should definitely be the bedroom. The bedroom will be easier to clean, and it can be made into a retreat from the world of allergenic substances.

How is a bedroom made allergy free?

The following are simple practical suggestions:

WALLS: The walls should be covered with wood panelling or an intact painted surface. Wallpaper is bad because it flakes as it ages and moulds grow in the paste under the paper. This is a particular problem if humidifiers and vaporizers have been used to excess. Fabric wall coverings such as hessian, or textured wallpapers are most undesirable. No pictures, pennants, bulletin or chalk boards should be in the room. The walls and ceiling should be wiped clean at least every 3 or 4 months.

WINDOWS: Smooth draperies, curtains or shades are best. Shutters, venetian blinds, corduroy or rough fabrics and ruffles are all dust collectors and not advisable. Heavy non-washable draperies should be blown free of dust in the dryer at least bimonthly. The windows should be kept closed at all times.

FLOORS: Tile or linoleum is best. Wood is preferable to carpeting of *any* type because all rugs retain dust. The exposed portions of wall-to-wall carpeting, regardless of the type, should be covered with non-skid plastic or linoleum. Daily vacuuming is not sufficient.

Young children need bare floors upon which to play. If the floors are cold, baseboard accessory electric heating might help. Allergic children should wear bed socks at night so that they do not directly touch the cold floor in the morning. There should be a small washable scatter rug at the bedside.

FURNITURE: This should be wooden, plastic or metal, simple in design, and never ornately carved. If upholstered, the covering should be smooth nylon, cotton, or plastic. The stuffing should be synthetic. Old upholstered or antique furniture often causes allergies. The room should be bare and contain as few pieces of furniture as possible.

BED: The headboard should not contain shelves unless they are empty. Canopy beds are dusty and not advisable. Extra beds in a room must be as allergy-free as the patients. If bunkbeds are used, the patient should sleep on the top. No storage should be allowed under the bed. Patients must sleep or nap only in their own room and own bed.

MATTRESS: This should be composed of synthetic foam or foam rubber; the latter should be checked to be certain that it does not smell mouldy. Polyurethane may have a strong irritating odour at times, and this can cause symptoms in some individuals. Mattresses must not be filled with kapok, disintegrating cotton, straw or horse hair. Old mouldy mattresses (due to bed wetting) should be replaced.

All types of mattresses must be *entirely* encased in plastic because any type can become dusty. Complete zippered plastic mattress covers are available or two fitted plastic covers can be used, one over the top and the other over the bottom.

Effective, inexpensive covers can be made by purchasing heavy gauge plastic sheeting or drop cloth material. These can be stapled or taped over the ends and bottoms of the mattress and box spring to encase them. Patients must be cautioned to replace or repair dry or cracked covers which are damaged by use. The mattress encasing may be covered by a *synthetic non-allergic* mattress pad or several fitted cotton sheets to decrease the discomfort of sleeping on plastic. Because mites (See page 142) are found on mattresses, the plastic top covering should be wiped clean each week when the linens are changed.

BOX SPRINGS: It should be entirely encased in plastic. Cotton covers are not dustproof. Children tend to bounce upon beds and if the mattress and box springs are not entirely encased, the dust can be shaken into the bedroom air.

PILLOWS: These should be synthetic, made of dacron, polyurethane, foam rubber or acrylon and washed every two weeks. Feathers, down, cotton, kapok, hair, wool or any disintegrating substance are not recommended. Synthetic or rubber pillows can break down to a dusty granular powder as they become older, and cause allergies. Foam rubber can become contaminated with mould spores or mites.

BEDSPREAD: It should be made of smooth fabric and be simple in design. There should be no ruffles or skirt.

BLANKETS: These should be cotton or synthetic and not fuzzy. Comforters must be filled with non-allergic material, *never feathers* kapok or hair. Blankets should be washed every two weeks.

DRESSER: This should not be cluttered. A simple shaded lamp, clock, radio or television are allowed providing they are dusted each day.

CHAIR: These should be simple, wooden or metal, and not upsholstered. The outside, if upholstered, should be plastic, cotton or nylon, and the inside filled with synthetic material

BOOKSHELVES: These should be empty and dusted often unless enclosed by sliding doors.

DESK: The top should be bare except for daily school material.

TOYS: Keep them in a tightly covered toy box or in enclosed drawers. Sporting goods should not be sitting in corners. Toys should be washable plastic, wood or metal. Stuffed toys must be examined to be certain they do not contain wool, kapok, feathers, disintegrating substances or hair. Burning a small amount of the outer cover and inside in an ashtray will reveal if it is composed of any animal material. The latter smells like a singed chicken when it is burned. The stuffing should not smell musty or mouldy. Play should be encouraged in the child's bedroom whenever possible.

CLOTHES CUPBOARD: This should contain only clothing worn at the present time. No storage of any type (shoe boxes, garment bags, etc.) should be permitted. The odour of cedar or mothballs is a problem for some allergic persons.

CLUTTER: Collections, such as cosmetics or games should not be kept in the bedroom unless they can be kept in an enclosed area or dresser drawer. The room should be stripped of all knick knacks or non-essentials.

CLEANING: Initially, and every three months, the room must be cleaned from the ceiling to the floor. Each item of furniture must be cleaned top, bottom, ends and sides. The floor should be cleaned thoroughly at least each week or two, and daily dusting is essential if daily symptoms are a problem. Dusting twice a week is indicated if symptoms occur 2 or 3 times weekly. Allergic persons should not assist or be present when the room is being cleaned or dusted. If an allergic person must clean, a special mask should be worn.

For daily dusting use a nylon dust mop which has a washable end piece, or a treated dust mop. Nylon develops static electricity and dust sticks completely to the mop and it cannot be shaken but must be washed off. Allergy dust inhibitors are available which can be used to diminish dust in carpets, drapes, furniture or bedding.

Some persons are worse on the day when their room is cleaned. This can happen if brooms or dusters, which tend to stir up dust are used. Vacuum cleaners can be checked in a dark room by running a flashlight along the seams and area where the bag is attached to see if any dust leaks are present.

Odourous substances should not be used to maintain an allergic person's bedroom. These include waxes, polishes, ammonia or oil. Reports concerning the allergenicity of various cleaning materials, medicinal sprays or insect repellent strips are scanty. Lysol contains phenol and can cause difficulty in some patients. Camphor, moth balls, insecticides, perfume and other strong smelling substances should be avoided.

The windows and the doors should be kept closed. Automatic door closers are often needed for small children who tend to run in and out of their rooms. Window fans are to be avoided because they can draw pollen and outside pollutants into the room.

Various types of air filters (See pages 151-156) are sometimes effective in eliminating major allergenic substances from bedroom atmospheres.

MITES: Most homes throughout the world are contaminated with invisible house dust mites. Live or dead mites, or their excreta are allergenic and are a major cause of house dust allergy. Mites grow best in a damp temperate climate at 25° to 30° C. They feed on human skin scales and food particles. The more mites in someone's home, the worse the allergies may be. Mites are found in and on mattresses, stuffed furniture, chairs, floors and clothing. The most important cause of allergy in bedroom dust is the mite. A warm bed, human scales from skin, and a high humidity are what mites particularly like. Keeping the home dry and vacuuming floors, mattresses and furniture will and often can help to diminish their numbers. Cleaning the tops of mattresses in particular should be helpful and blankets and bedding should be washed often. Exposure to sunlight decreases the number of mites. Mites on clothing can be killed during washing. A safe effective chemical or spray is not known at the present time which kills mites.

Mites are also found in cereal grains, cheese, on birds, in birdcages and in household dust everywhere in the world.

Persons allergic to house dust are sometimes significantly helped if treated with mite extract injections.

MISCELLANEOUS: The presence of flowers, plants, and smoking within an allergic person's bedroom is not advisable. Do not plant trees directly outside the window. If they cannot be removed, inform your allergist so that your treatment extract can be appropriately adjusted.

What causes allergies in the living or family room?

Recommendations made in relation to the bedroom, also apply to the living or family room. Give special attention to the room where the patient spends or plays much of the time. Special problems related to these rooms are as follows:

FLOORS: Small children tend to play on the floor with toys and to watch television lying on their belly. For this reason, wood, tile, or linoleum, which can be kept relatively dust-free, are best. Carpeting of *any type* is dusty and can cause allergies. Woollen carpeting is bad because the wool (and possibly moths) can be additional causes of allergy. Vacuum the family or living room carpet daily. Discourage sitting *directly on* the carpet and encourage sitting on wooden furniture. The carpet should be covered with skid-proof plastic or one small area covered with a piece of linoleum, plastic or a washable cotton blanket. Children can be told this is their magic carpet and they are not allowed on the rest of the carpet which can become dusty. Confine floor play to the special covered carpeted area.

FURNITURE: Ideally, furniture should have a smooth cotton or nylon (not wool or mohair) covering and the stuffing should be a synthetic or rubber product. Kapok, down or feathers, animal hair and cotton stuffing are not advisable. Stuffed furniture should be vacuumed daily and torn or damaged pieces must be repaired or replaced. Check toss pillows to be certain the filling is synthetic and not disintegrated. If the furniture has a cover, clean it frequently and vacuum the fabric underneath the cover.

FLOWERS: Fresh flowers cause allergies because heavy pollen is shaken from them as they are arranged or moved. Dried flowers can be contaminated with mould spores. Artificial flowers need cleaning because they become dusty. Smelling roses can cause sneezing in grass sensitive patients if grass pollen has blown onto them. Ragweed pollen sensitive persons often have difficulty from exposure to daisies, marigolds, chrysanthemums and zinnias.

What causes allergies in kitchens?

Symptoms of allergies are caused mainly by eating a food or the odour of a raw or cooked food. Sifting flour, cracking an egg or opening a jar of peanut butter can all cause sudden symptoms in some patients. The taste or odour of the following foods may cause symptoms: nuts, fish, white potatoes, fresh fruit, chocolate, eggs, peanut butter or milk.

The kitchen is considered to be one of the least allergenic areas in the house. Kitchen aerosols, gas fumes, carpeting or improperly functioning exhaust fans above stoves can all cause symptoms in some individuals.

What causes allergies in the bathroom?

The two major offenders are mould spores and perfumed substances. The latter includes soaps, bubble baths, body powders or lotions, oils or creams, after-shaving lotions, hair sprays, bathroom aerosols, hair oils, scented facial or toilet tissues and underarm deodorants.

Other potential causes of allergy are: tooth powders, brushes (hair or tooth) made from animal hair, and dust or moulds in carpeting. In particular, check for moulds in the shower stall area. (See page 147).

Cleaning solutions or paint used on toilet seats can cause a rash on the upper thighs and lower buttocks, in the area which comes in contact with the seat. Plastic seats are preferable.

What causes allergies in basements or the crawl space under homes?

Dust and moulds are major offenders. Cleaning and dusting a basement often precipitates allergic symptoms in sensitive individuals. This can be diminished by wearing a special mask. (See page 261). Clothes dryers should be vented properly to help reduce dust and lint. Clothing dried in a damp, musty basement can acquire a musty smell which could cause symptoms. If clothes are not immediately dried after washing, they can smell mouldy or musty. (See page 152 concerning problems related to furnaces.)

What causes allergies in cars?

Cars cause allergy symptoms because of cigarette smoke, animal hair and air pollution. Cars are often dusty and not well-cleaned. Inside floor mats and upholstery should be vacuumed regularly and the metal inside should be washed. Car pillows should be synthetic. Open convertible cars acquire a lasting mouldy odour if they are accidentally open during a rainstorm. (See page 147).

Tinted glass is helpful to reduce nose symptoms triggered by sunlight. Air conditioners aid in decreasing pollen and air pollution. Draughts from open windows can sometimes cause nose symptoms.

Sudden allergic symptoms can occur while travelling. After several to many miles the problems just as suddenly disappear. Sometimes this happens each time a certain area is passed because of some airborne allergenic or irritating substance in that region. At other times it is a seasonal problem due to some item which is pollinating at that time of the year or some factory which is temporarily polluting the atmosphere with an offensive substance. Recent road construction chemicals also can be at fault.

Which hobbies cause allergies?
   This list could be as long as the list of hobbies. A few major ones are: gardening (moulds, sprays, herbicides and insecticides), sewing or knitting (animal hair) printing (flaxseed – wet newsprint), pets (hair, dandruff and saliva), music (composition of mouth pieces or resin on bows), paints or woodwork, decorations or art work (hay or straw), gourmet cooking (dried herbs or roots), camping (sleeping bags should be synthetic, never down, cotton or kapok), judo or wrestling on dusty mats.

Can glue cause allergy?
   Fish glue can. It is usually caramel coloured. Licking stamps, envelopes, stickers, contact glued boxes, book bindings, toys, or even old furniture can cause symptoms. White coloured paste seldom causes difficulty. Clear colourless glue and cements used for model aeroplanes can cause symptoms because of their odour.

Does paint cause allergies?
   It certainly can. *Alkyd* paints are least allergenic. These are "non-odorous". They do not have any mineral solvents so the paint brush can be cleaned with water. The odour which they produce is mainly due to the pigment. Other so-called "odourless" paints are oil-based and the aroma is due to the "odourless" solvent. If they are used in poorly ventilated areas, the fumes can sometimes be toxic. Linseed oil used in some paints causes difficulty in some allergic persons. Rubber based paints are seldom used at the present time. The odour from these can last for months. Some individuals are sensitive to the turpentine or mineral spirit smell. If paint causes symptoms, avoid it.
   Try to paint during the warm months. If paint causes symptoms, avoid direct or indirect contact with the freshly painted areas until the odour is gone. This may entail staying with friends or relatives temporarily. The odour of most household paints is eliminated in a few days, seldom more than a week, *if* the area is well-ventilated at room temperature (20° to 27° C). If the area is not well-ventilated, paint odours may last for a month or so.

OUTDOORS

What causes allergies in the area of your home?
   Grasses cause allergy mainly when they pollinate (See page 260). If grass is cut very short and often, fewer symptoms will be noticed because the top of the grass will not grow long enough to develop pollen before it is cut. Children have symptoms when they play on lawns or touch balls which roll on the grass.
   Symptoms can occur from cutting grass because this shakes grass pollen into the air.

In areas where snow is a problem, grass moulds can cause symptoms, especially when the snow is melting. Fallen trees can also become mouldy. Youngsters playing ball have symptoms because moulds adhere to the ball surface.

Lawn maintenance, includes seeding, fertilizing and using herbicides, all have been known to cause mild to severe allergic symptoms.

Landscaping – In general, flowers do not cause allergic symptoms, unless they are held close to the face. Problems arise when someone picks flowers and sniffs them, or when adults or older children help maintain the home border by removing weeds. Moulds can contaminate both soil and plants. Garden sprays and insecticides can cause allergies.

Trees – The trees which cause most symptoms are the ones which lose their leaves every year. Just before the warm season begins there are little flowers, which are barely visible. They produce pollen for a period of one to several weeks, which can blow for many miles. Trees located close to a patient's bedroom window often cause symptoms. Some trees, such as fruit trees, have large and colourful flowers, but do not cause allergies because insects spread the pollen rather than the wind. Raking leaves or playing in leaf piles can cause symptoms because of moulds which are found on them.

Air Pollution – Studies are being carried out in many areas of the world in relation to allergies and air pollution. It is possible for some factory contaminants to precipitate allergic symptoms immediately or several hours after exposure. Community large scale insecticide use to eradicate flies or to spray orchards or food crops can cause symptoms. Persons who have allergies should notice if certain odours, thermal inversions, or types of pollution are related to their symptoms.

HOUSE DUST

What is house dust?

House dust consists of disintegrated fibres, cellulose, organic material, mites (See page 142), cotton, kapok, feathers, furniture stuffing, lint, draperies, rugs, rug pads, mohair, wool, moulds, food particles, insecticides, bacteria, insects, animal hair, and dandruff. Insect hair, excrement, eggs and decomposed or live bodies of ants, bees, beetles, cocoons, cockroaches, flies, mites, moths, and mosquitos can cause allergy. Outside dirt, unless it is mouldy, is not the cause of allergies.

How can you detect a house dust allergy?

The easiest way would be to notice if exposure to dust for example, dusting furniture or emptying the vacuum cleaner causes allergy. Prophylactically dust sensitive persons are sometimes helped by using a special "mask" (See page 261) to limit dust contact during cleaning.

MOULDS

Can mould contamination within a home be identified?
A mildew odour is often obvious, although it is possible to become so accustomed to the smell that it is not noticed. Culture and identification of mould spores within a home can be done with a doctor's supervision. Commonly contaminated areas are damp, dark places, such as cellars, attics, store rooms, crawl spaces beneath homes, food cellars, greenhouses, bathrooms and shower areas.

How can mould contamination be diminished?
1. Moulds grow best in a high humidity. Dehumidifiers remove enormous quantities of moisture. These machines can substantially control mould growth. Parents should not use humidifiers or room vaporizers in excess, in children's rooms.
2. Mould contaminated items must be removed or cleaned with chemicals to stop mould growth. Awnings, blankets, camping equipment, carpets, draperies, firewood, floors, foam rubber products, leather goods, mattresses, paper items (books), rubber gaskets, sealing refrigerator doors, shades, shoes and upholstery can all be contaminated. Children's winter boots are often mouldy. Plants within homes can be contaminated, as can aquariums.
3. Foods which can be mouldy would include cheese, dried or candied fruit, melons, mushrooms, soy sauce, steaks (aged) smoked or pickled products, wine and beer.
4. Basement and cellar cracks which allow mould (See page 144) must be repaired. Silicone-rubber sealers effectively fill in the cracks. Basements should be lighted and well-ventilated. Keep windows open during the warm months unless this interferes with the dehumidifier. Homes with dirt floors, crawl spaces, or without damp courses are often heavily contaminated.
5. Thoroughly clean mildewy surfaces which cannot be replaced with a mould resistant cleaning preparation.
Bathrooms or damp areas should be painted with a mould resistant paint. Mouldy wallpaper should be removed and the walls painted or panelled.
6. Moisture can accumulate in air-conditioners. (See page 155).
7. Some furnace and room air purifiers remove mould spores from the air (See page 151).

Do mould spores outside your home cause allergies?
Mould spores are in the air in high concentrations at certain times of the year in many parts of the world. Fewer moulds are found in dry areas with high altitudes. Vegetation at the end of the warm

season, is often contaminated with moulds, as are grains, leaves from trees, straw, hay, tree bark and soil. High concentrations of mould spores are on all cereal crops when they are ripe, so harvesting grain is not advisable for mould allergic patients.

Are patients helped if their home is allergy-free?

Patients are helped if they are sensitive to something within their home and they have followed suggestions made on pages 137 to 156. The symptoms should diminish or subside within 2 to 4 weeks. It is amazing, however, how often after thorough explanation and detailed written instructions a home is still not reasonably allergy-free. The degree of thoroughness with which you carry out the suggestions made by your allergist is often directly related to the amount of improvement that you will notice.

If home changes are made properly it may be possible to prevent or delay the necessity for skin testing and extract therapy in some patients.

Some patients have a choice. Their symptoms can be relieved to a significant degree by changing their home, diet, or by receiving allergy injection therapy. Surprisingly some patients prefer injection treatments. Other patients have little choice. Their allergies are so severe that they require the combined beneficial effect of home and dietary changes, *plus* injection therapy before satisfactory strides are made towards improvement in their health.

HUMIDITY

How is humidity related to allergy?

The mucous membranes of the breathing passageways which includes the lining of the lungs, nose and sinuses must be moist. Little hairs in these areas move a thin layer of mucous and inhaled material continually towards the throat. If the breathing tract is not moist, the little hairs will not function properly. This can lead to breathing problems and a proneness to infection. Inadequate humidification can contribute to excessive mouth and skin dryness and itching, in particular in eczema patients.

Dust settles in rooms with a normal humidity but floats in the air in a dry atmosphere.

What should be the humidity in a home?

The usual recommended level is forty to fifty per cent when the indoor temperature is 20° C. Practically, however, if the outside temperature is zero, a home relative humidity of 25 per cent is recommended. If the temperature is minus 6.7° C. or above outside, the home humidity should be about 35 per cent. Lower room temperatures are more tolerable if humidification is adequate. Many homes tend to be too dry during the colder months, requiring additional humidification; and too moist in the warm weather, requiring some means of dehumidification.

What is relative humidity?
This is the amount of moisture in the air compared to the amount of moisture the air can hold at a given temperature.

How can relative humidity be measured?
Shops sell instruments which measure humidity in much the same way as a thermometer will measure one's temperature. Each room should be individually checked because there may be some variation in humidity.

TEMPERATURE

What is the optimal temperature for a person's bedroom?
Although there are personal preferences, the bedroom temperature should not be lower than 18.3° – 20° C. If a room is too hot or too cold, or the temperature changes quickly, some patients suddenly develop allergic symptoms. The suggested optimal temperature is 21.1° – 22.2° C.

HEATING YOUR HOME

Which type of heating is best?
Unfortunately, there is no uniform opinion among allergists concerning this most important point. Electric heat does not pollute the air but it is expensive in some countries and in some homes, impractical. All types of heating have advantages and disadvantages. The choice often depends upon where a person happens to live, what is available in that area, or which type of heating a family can afford.
A fairly large number of allergists recommend a forced hot air heating system with a central air-conditioner, humidifier and furnace air-purifier. Realistically, however, this is a very expensive way of heating a home. A compromise which might be almost as effective would be to install an air-conditioner and an air-purifier in the bedroom of the person who has allergies. If an air-conditioner is too expensive, a large circulating fan might be helpful.

What are the disadvantages of a forced hot air heating system?
This form of heat is drying and supplementary humidification is essential. A blower in the furnace will move the warm air throughout the house, but this will circulate particles of dust and other allergenic substances. Filters, placed at the furnace outlet, are beneficial if they are

cleaned or replaced regularly. Many people do not know that their filter should be cleaned monthly.

There are two main types of furnace filters. One which costs relatively little, is used for about a month and is discarded. A second so-called "permanent" type costs more, but lasts for long periods of time and can be washed whenever necessary. You can determine when a filter needs cleaning by looking at it. In general, a 4 week schedule seems best although some filters may need cleaning every week or two. Inadequate filter care not only contributes to allergic problems, but can interfere with heat distribution and increase home heating costs.

The duct work from the furnace can become dusty and although air is filtered as it leaves the furnace, it can pick up dust as it passes through the ducts. This dust then can be blown throughout the house. If the duct work is dusty, it may have to be cleaned.

One other disadvantage to a forced hot-air heating system is that air pollution is produced from either gas or oil heat. Gas is not pure, so when it is burned, it produces more than water and carbon dioxide. Natural gas can produce offensive sulphur dioxide. Combustion products do not always escape to the outside because of back draughts and leaks between the combustion and warm air chambers. There is even some suggestion that leaking raw gas from any gas appliance can contribute to allergies. The smell and combustion of oil, used for heating likewise is sometimes thought to aggravate allergies.

If a forced hot-air heating system is used in a home in conjunction with a furnace air-purifying system, it is essential that the furnace blower be adjusted so that it is constantly in use throughout the year even though this can cause a cool draught. If this is not done, the air will not be circulated frequently enough to allow for maximum cleaning. Normally, the furnace blower is adjusted so that it is utilized only when the thermostat indicates that heat is necessary.

What are the advantages and disadvantages of steam or water heat?

This type of heat is sometimes recommended by allergists. The heating units should be accessible for thorough cleaning. Electric steam heat does not contaminate the air in contrast to gas or oil steam heat. It is, however, more expensive than other water heating methods, and not always available. It provides no method for removal of dust or pollen from the atmosphere. As with hot air heat, it is drying and supplementary humidification may be required.

Is radiant heat beneficial?

Some allergists believe this is the best type of heat for allergic persons. It is, however, relatively expensive. The floor type of radiant heat is not practical because the concrete slab which contains heat within copper or iron pipes tends to heat and cool slowly over a period of hours. The pipes can deteriorate and leak. Within the concrete mass it is difficult to find the exact point of deterioration. Floor radiant heat can only be used in homes which have a basement. There is a ceiling type of radiant heat, but this keeps the ceiling unduly warm while the lower parts of the room may be cool. A major advantage of radiant heat is that it does not pollute the air. It, however, provides no method of removing dust or pollen and requires extra humidification.

Do space heaters cause allergies?
This type of heat is often used in older or rural homes, or in warm countries where a source of heat is seldom required. Air pollution will be caused by whatever type of fuel is burned to supply the heat. Formaldehyde, a non-specific irritant, can also be produced by oil space heaters. Supplementary heat is often required in certain rooms because of poorly balanced heating systems. In these situations electric heat is least apt to contaminate the air.

AIR-CLEANERS

How effective is air purification?
Portable machines are said to circulate room air approximately two to ten times per hour depending upon the room size and type and capacity of the machine. Most companies claim that 95 per cent of all airborne particles and up to 99 per cent of all pollens are removed. Bacteria ranging in diameter from 0.1 to 10 microns* and smoke ranging from 0.1 to 1.0 micron in size are also removed. Most antigenic pollen is in the 15 to 30 micron size, while mould spores range from 1.0 to 40 microns.

Which types of air purifiers are available?
The answer depends upon where you live. Purifiers can electronically remove allergenic particles. Others called HEPA filters push the air through special glass fibre pieces which sift the air and remove particles down to the 0.1 micron range. HEPA is an abbreviation for high efficiency particulate air filter.

Does air purification help patients who have allergies?
Although many patients and physicians are favourably impressed with air purifiers, few scientific medical confirmatory studies are presently available. Dramatic and almost overnight improvement can be noted in some persons, however, after this machine is placed in their bedroom. Other allergic persons do not find these machines helpful in
* Human hair is about 65 microns in diameter.

any way. Unquestionably bedrooms are most "allergy-free" when the
units are properly cleaned and used.

Where can air-purifiers be obtained?

Furnace units are handled by furnace specialists who also install air-
conditioning systems. Some units are sold through suppliers of electrical
goods or large department stores.

Is a furnace or room unit best?

Both have advantages and disadvantages. A room unit of the proper
size can keep a room so clean that no visible dust accumulates on furniture. It is portable. It helps, however, only when the patient is in that
particular room. Some of these units are noisy and can interfere with the
sleep.

Room air-purifiers are helpful if a person travels because they are
portable and can be used in any bedroom.

Electronic furnace units help to make an entire home more "allergy-
free". During the warmer months, however, a furnace air-conditioner is
essential for comfort because the doors and windows should be kept
closed at all times. During the winter months the furnace blower must be
utilized constantly to keep the air circulating and clean. Central heating
systems ideally, are supposed to heat all rooms equally and well. In
reality, however, a balanced heating system is a rarity. Most homes have
some rooms which are heated well and others poorly. If an electronic
air-purifying system is installed in the furnace, these same rooms would
therefore have varying degrees of air purification. A furnace unit,
however, would definitely be preferable if several members of a family
had allergies.

Another problem is that a furnace installation is possible only in
homes which have a forced hot air heating system. Homes heated by
other means, will not have ducts for circulating air so the cost of separate
ductwork for air purifying and cooling is often prohibitive.

How costly are air-purifiers?

The price varies depending on the brand of machine and the country
in which it were sold. In general, the units are relatively expensive.

Where in a room should the machine be placed?

The machines must be placed a few inches away from the wall because
air needs to circulate behind and through some of the machines. The
machines should not blow air into the patient's face because the
machines produce a distinct, cool draught. It is better if the air blows indirectly towards the patients so they breathe clean air but have no
draught. Electronic machines cause a peculiar sparking noise which

often indicates the machine needs cleaning. If the electric or HEPA machine produces a strong offensive odour, the machine should be checked by the distributor.

How should the room electronic air-purifiers be cleaned?
Read and carefully follow the specific directions which accompany each machine concerning care and cleaning. The machines will *not* help if used improperly. If dust is noted on the furniture it often indicates that the machine either needs cleaning or it is not functioning properly.

How can you tell if a machine will remove pollen?
Blow smoke through the machine. Smoke particles are smaller than pollen. If the machine effectively removes these smaller particles, it definitely would remove pollen particles.

What is the ozone odour noted with some electrostatic air cleaning machines?
Ozone is a special form of oxygen which has a peculiar characteristic odour. New machines sometimes produce a relatively large amount of ozone but this diminishes after a few days. If it does not, the machine should be returned. Most people find the slight odour of ozone refreshing, but there are some individuals who are very sensitive to the slightest amount and find it very irritating. This type of individual may not be able to use this type of machine but possibly might be helped by a HEPA filter which never produces ozone.

Air purifiers may have a charcoal impregnated filter to reduce the amount of ozone which the machine produces or to eliminate odours. Ozone production increases with decreasing humidity.

If a machine produces excessive amounts of ozone, you would quickly become aware of it because it could cause shortness of breath, a dry cough, irritation and watering of the eyes and nose. If these problems are noted, the machine should not be used.

Ozone production is not confined entirely to machines. In some cities where smog is a problem there is a type of photochemical air pollution which can produce such high ozone concentrations that symptoms are produced.

Should this machine be used throughout the day?
The recommendations would vary depending upon the patient. If a person were doing well, it might be adequate to use such a machine only 12 hours a day. Others need it 24 hours a day. If the machine's sound were an annoyance, use the machine during the day. If the machine were used 12 hours a day in a bedroom, it could be utilized in some other room during the night.

A common misconception is that the machine is useful only when the allergic person is in that particular room. The machine can cleanse the air whether someone is in the room or not.

Do air-purifying machines help if windows and doors are open?
If a large amount of pollution is continually entering a room from the outside, the machine would obviously not work as effectively as it might otherwise. To produce truly clean room air, the same air must remain in the room so that the machine can eventually thoroughly clean it.

If a room becomes too warm because the windows are closed and a fan is not helpful, the machine should be used 24 hours a day and the windows opened. Place the machine so the clean air leaving it blows indirectly towards the patient's head. In this way a draught is avoided but clean air is inhaled.

When should a bedroom be aired out?
This is best done during the middle of the day rather than in the early morning hours or late at night.

AIR-CONDITIONERS

How helpful are air-conditioners for allergies?
Many allergic children or adults are relieved of their symptoms when they are in an air-conditioned area. Others, however, surprisingly instantly become worse. This individual variation is poorly understood. Before an air-conditioner is purchased, be certain that this machine does not have an undesirable effect.

The major function of air-conditioners is to cool and remove moisture from the air. Most also contain some type of filtering system which should be beneficial for larger air particles.

Is an automobile air-conditioner helpful?
These machines can filter out pollen and road dust. Because the windows are closed during use, pollens and air pollutants cannot blow into the car.

Do air-conditioners remove pollen?
There are many misleading and confusing claims in regard to pollen and dust removal. Air-conditioners often contain a mechanical or impingement filter which is in essence like a fine screen. The size particle which it removes would depend upon the size, composition and quality of the mechanical filter. Large dust particles and pollens may be removed by high quality fibrous filters. Some claim that a standard air-conditioner filter is about 80 per cent efficient in trapping particles

approximately 20 microns in size. If an air-conditioner were used in a closed room recirculating the air, it is possible that this machine would be effective for some patients. The problem, however, is that 90 per cent of airborne particles are 5 microns or less and ordinary air-conditioners supposedly would not be able to filter out these smaller dust particles, mould spores or smoke. Patients who are sensitive to small particles of this size would need more efficient electronic or HEPA air purifiers.

Do air-conditioners cause allergies?

Under certain circumstances they could. Because they dehumidify as well as cool, some are contaminated with mould spores. The typical odour of mould may be obvious when they are used initially at the onset of the warm season. If a mouldy odour is noticed, all washable parts should be washed or sprayed with a mould resistant solution. (See page 147).

Are there different types of air-conditioners?

There is one type of air-conditioner which only recirculates the air within a room while cooling and dehumidifying it. Other more expensive or larger types, also ventilate or exchange about 10 per cent of the room air with the outside air. This latter type could circulate pollen during certain seasons and possibly aggravate a person's allergic symptoms. Machines which bring in fresh air have a switch indicating *ventilate* or *fresh air*. This switch should be kept in the "off" position and only the "recirculate" indicator should be used. Exhaust and fresh air vents should not be used.

What is the most inexpensive way to make a room allergy-free and comfortable?

The room should be thoroughly cleaned and contain as little furniture as possible. There should be no carpet, the mattress and box spring should be encased in plastic, and the pillows should be synthetic. The room should have an air purifier and if the room tends to be too warm, a fan can be installed or if this is not satisfactory a room air-conditioner could be utilized. A room humidifier might be desirable but is not essential for most patients.

Can air-conditioners and humidifiers cause respiratory problems?

A disease called a hypersensitivity pneumonitis has been traced to contamination of air-conditioners and humidifiers in offices and homes. The organism which causes the difficulty is often a mould spore. Nose symptoms can persist for a long time before chills, fever, coughing and shortness of breath are noticed. Prolonged exposure to contaminated equipment can cause progressive fatigue and weight loss. The X-ray sometimes reveals changes. Patients who suspect this problem should check with their physician. The air-conditioner or humidifier can be examined as well as the patient's blood. Skin tests do not show an immediate reaction. The sudden occurrence of symptoms is sometimes noted 4 to 6 hours after exposure to contaminated equipment. It is possible to be well on weekends if the problem is related to an air-conditioner at work, and to be sick while co-workers might have similar complaints and health problems at work. If the contaminated machines were in your home, you would feel ill only when you were at home.

Cortisone and disodium cromoglycate help patients who have this problem, while antibiotics do not. The best way to eliminate this problem, is to separate the patient from exposure to the source of his problem. Either remove the organism from the contaminated air-conditioner or humidifier, or seek a different place of employment if the problem occurs only at work.

MOVING

What advice might help when your family moves?
If your family is considering a move to a nearby new home, consider the allergic potential of the new home to which you are moving as suggested on page 138. If the allergic individual must have contact with dusty stored items, a dust mask (See page 261) should be worn and either asthma or hay fever drugs taken to prevent attacks. Allergic children, if possible, should not be home when the actual moving takes place and should not assist in preparatory packing and cleaning. If the new home needs repainting, this should be done prior to the move.

How is allergy treatment continued after a distant move?
1.   If you are receiving allergy extract therapy, obtain an extract injection treatment a day prior to the actual move, even if it is not needed. A new home in a new area can cause an extremely busy time and it is easy to forget an allergy extract treatment. If treatment were received just prior to the move, another won't be due for several weeks. By then the family should be settled in the new home.
2.   Prior to your move to a new section of the country, check with your allergist about future allergy treatments. Your allergist may want to continue to care for you personally by seeing you at infrequent but regular intervals. If the services of a different allergist who lived closer to the area in which you moved would be desirable, your present allergist can help determine who should be seen.

If you change allergists, send a letter to your previous allergist stating that your records should be sent to the new physician.

Sometimes a child or adult first begins an allergy evaluation a short period of time prior to a move. While it may be essential to secure immediate advice about allergies, it probably would be best if skin testing were delayed until after the move to the new area. The physician who does allergy skin testing and advises about extract therapy should *whenever possible* be the same physician who is going to provide prolonged personal allergy care. Most allergists would prefer personally to carry out a thorough evaluation in their own individual manner only for patients who are to be under their care for many years. A new patient who has never been evaluated for his allergies is much less complicated and often can be helped more quickly and easily than a patient transferred from another physician.

A major consideration, however, may be the availability of an allergy specialist. Some countries have only a few who are located mainly in large cities. The selection may be quite limited.

CHAPTER TWELVE

Detecting food allergy

How can you tell if you have a food allergy?
If a food is causing a symptom, it should disappear when the food is not eaten and reappear when that food is again eaten.

Foods can be related to a symptom which was not thought to be due to allergies. A patient on a milk-free diet to relieve asthma, might find that his asthma would not be helped, but that his disposition, nose symptoms, or frequent headaches stop.

Foods which cause immediate problems are easy to detect (although they might be quite difficult to avoid because of poor labelling of pre-packaged foods). Foods, such as milk and wheat, may not cause symptoms for several hours (6 - 24) after eating making it much more difficult to figure out the cause.

It is possible for an adult to have an intestinal, nose, or chest problem start as a food allergy in infancy and persist and bother him his whole life. Many adults are unaware that they have a food allergy. Some patients have digestive problems as their *ONLY* manifestation of allergy and the correct diagnosis is missed for years because there are so many other more common causes of digestive complaints.

Which parts of the body can be affected by food allergy?
Food allergy can cause many types of symptoms.

A.   Common areas of the body which are affected are:

SKIN:
Itching of any part of body
   skin
Welts or nettle rash – look
   like mosquito bites
Eczema – rash in creases of
   arms or legs — or all over
Body swelling – face, joints,
   fingers — any body area

CHEST:
Coughing
Wheezing
Excess mucus in lungs
Rattle in chest

158

NOSE:
Sneezing several times in
   a row
Runny watery mucus
Stuffy nose
Itching (nose rubbing or
   wiggling)
Throat-clearing
Snorting nose sounds

INTESTINES:
Diarrhoea or constipation
Upset stomach
Bellyache or cramps
Nausea or vomiting – colic
   in infants (See page 84)
Excess mucus or gas
Bloating
Poor appetite

EYES:
Itching, redness, watery
   mucus
Puffy eyes
Dark circles under
   eyes

B.   Less common manifestations of food allergies affect:

EARS:
Recurrent fluid formation behind ear drums.

BRAIN:
Headaches
Body or muscle aches
Disposition changes,
   irritability, or
   behaviour problems

Hyperactivity
Fatigue—tension
Convulsions
Shock

C.   Very rare forms of allergy which seldom are associated with eating certain foods can be:

LIPS:
Scaling, red, or swollen

MOUTH:
Repeated cold sores, canker sores
   or bad breath odours

GENITALS:
Itching or rash of
   genital or rectal area

It is possible for a food item to produce one of the above symptoms, for dust to produce another, and for pollen to cause a third. Remember that *many* diseases unrelated to allergy can cause similar symptoms. A physician will help you confirm any suspicion you have about food allergy.

Do special foods tend to cause selected symptoms?

Certain foods are somewhat more common causes of some allergic problems than others. The listed foods are frequent (but NOT the only) causes of the following:

CHEST AND NOSE ALLERGIES	Milk, wheat, eggs, chocolate (cola or peanuts (peanut butter), corn
EAR ALLERGIES	Milk, peanuts, chocolate, corn
ECZEMA	Citrus, tomato, milk, egg, peanut
WELTS (NETTLE RASH) OR BODY SWELLING (ANGIOEDEMA)	Egg, pork, citrus, tomato, nuts, berries, fish, aspirin
INTESTINAL PROBLEMS	Milk, wheat, egg, apple, pea (peanuts, peanut butter)
TENSION AND FATIGUE HYPERACTIVITY	Milk, corn, chocolate (cola), tomato, potato, dyed food items
HEADACHE	Milk, chocolate (cola), corn, peanuts (peas), onions, garlic, pork, egg, cinnamon
CANKER SORES	Citrus, apple, vinegar, tomato, toothpaste, pineapple, banana, walnut, chocolate
BAD BREATH	Chocolate, egg.

Note that milk is the most common cause of food allergy.

(Table by kind permission of Dr. Frederic Speer)

At what age do people start to have food allergies?

Although infants are most frequently allergic to foods, food allergies can occur at any age. Many foods cause obvious symptoms during the first year of life but the allergy disappears within a year or two. Strong allergies, however, often persist throughout a lifetime. Adults who develop a food allergy may be unable to eat a certain food for a number of years, and then for no apparent reason lose that food sensitivity. If they are unfortunate they can acquire other food allergies as they lose their previous ones, or a food allergy which disappeared can recur.

Can food allergies be prevented during infancy?

For many years allergists have believed that the longer an infant was breast fed, the less likely that allergies would occur. It was strongly urged that infants not be fed highly allergenic foods such as eggs and chocolate early in life. To diminish the development of food allergies, mixed cereals should not be used. Rather give the baby rice on one day, barley the next, then oats, etc. (See Chapter 86). A recent study indicates that cow's milk causes allergy earlier in life, than breast milk. Soya milk is less allergenic than cow's milk. The overall rate of development of allergy, however, seems to be the same whether an infant is fed breast, cow's or soya milk. Infants of allergic parents are more apt to develop food allergy than babies born in families where allergies are not a problem.

How often does food cause allergies?

Food frequently causes infant allergies. It has been estimated that maybe 5 to 10 per cent of allergic children are sensitive to foods. This cause of allergy becomes less evident as children age because food allergies tend to be outgrown.

Food allergies are often seen in patients who have not outgrown their infantile eczema. Sometimes one allergy can disappear, while others are retained, throughout life. Occasionally, adults develop an acute allergy to a food which caused no allergic symptoms in the past. Alcohol in all forms, particularly champagne, can give rise to sudden nose and chest allergic symptoms.

Some allergists believe that food allergics are infrequent while others commonly diagnose this problem. The success in detection is often related to the degree of the allergist's interest. The more one investigates along these lines, the more food allergies one finds.

Why do food allergies develop?

Usually we don't know why they occur. A very young baby's intestines will allow incompletely digested foods to pass more readily into the blood stream. As the digestive system ages, only digested foods pass. This may be, in part, the reason for infant allergies decreasing as they get older. If foods are not well digested, they are more apt to cause an allergy to develop. The tendency to develop a new food allergy can occur during or shortly after the period when a patient has diarrhoea. Highly allergenic foods (See page 85), therefore, should be avoided shortly after a digestive upset or until the bowel movements seem to be normal.

Are all digestive problems due to allergies?

No. It is sometimes easy to be certain that a food is the cause of a symptom. This does *not*, however, mean that the person is allergic to that food. For example, it is possible for many people to have loose bowel movements or an excessive amount of intestinal gas after eating prunes or baked beans. This effect is unrelated to allergies. Some families of patients cannot eat greasy foods, certain cereal grains (gluten), or drink milk because they lack certain digestive enzymes. Certain milk sugars, for example, can cause constant diarrhoea in infants and adults on this basis. It is obviously possible for contaminated or spoiled foods to cause a belly upset which is not allergic. Improperly canned food products can have toxic substances in them which can cause illness. Patients who have fibrocystic disease will notice frothy, greasy, foul-smelling bowel movements. Many digestive problems in infants are due to the preparation or method of feeding. None of these problems should be thought to be due to allergies.

Which foods seldom cause allergy?
    See List III on page 163.
    In some patients, however, these foods do cause symptoms. For example, an infant switched from wheat to rice cereal to eliminate an allergic problem could eventually become allergic to rice. Rice is often not suspected because it is so infrequently a source of allergy.
    People in different countries eat different foods. Patients are most apt to become allergic to the foods which they frequently eat. If a person is raised in a country where large quantities of lamb rather than pork are eaten, that person would be more apt to be allergic to lamb than to pork. A person who does not eat any pork products for religious reasons would not be allergic to pork.

***After* the infant period which foods cause most allergies?**
    See List I on page 163. Fresh foods cause allergies sometimes only because of moulds or insecticides on the outside. Fresh fruits often cause immediate symptoms. Cooking foods alter foods proteins so that they are changed into forms which may or may not cause allergy. Canning foods has a similar effect but preservatives or artificial colouring or flavouring can contribute to an allergy.
    Flour can cause allergies when it is sifted and breathed. This is a common problem among bakers. Other patients have difficulty only when they eat foods which contain flour (wheat).

Are there varying degrees of food allergies?
    It is possible to be so allergic to milk, wheat, or eggs, for example, that none can be eaten in *any* form at *any* time. Patients who are not very sensitive might find they could tolerate these foods in baked goods, but could not eat them in their typical form. For example, eggs baked in cakes might be alright, but a soft-boiled egg might cause symptoms.
    When attempting to figure out a food allergy, the first problem is to determine whether a person is allergic to a particular food or not. The second problem is to decide how much of the offending food can be eaten without causing symptoms. There are patients who can drink one glass of milk a day, but if they take two, they have allergies. (See page 166 re thresholds.)

Which foods cause allergy?

I FOODS MOST OFTEN CAUSING ALLERGY	II FOODS SOMETIMES CAUSING ALLERGY	III FOODS SELDOM CAUSING ALLERGY
Bananas	Apples	Apricots & their Juice
Beans—Lima or Lentils	Beef	Bacon
Berries	Celery	Barley
Chocolate (Cola)	Citrus Fruits	Beets
Cinnamon	(After Infancy)	Carrots
Coconut	Cherries	Chicken (Male)
Corn	Chicken (Female)	Coffee
Diet Beverages	Colouring Agents	Cranberries & their
Egg White	Cottonseed	Juice
Fish—All Types	Food Colouring	Ginger Ale
Including Crab,	Garlic	Grapes & their Juice
Lobster & Shrimp	Melons	Green Beans
Iodized Salt	Mushrooms	Honey
Mayonnaise	Potatoes (White)	Lamb
Milk	Prunes	Oats
Monosodium	Spices	Peaches & their
Glutamate	Spinach	Juice
Mustard	Vinegar (Apple	Pears & their Juice
Nuts—Oil &	Cider)	Pineapples & their
Extracts	Vitamins	Juice
Orange or Citrus		Poi
(Especially during		Raisins
Infancy)		Rice
Peanut Butter		Rye
Peas		Salt
Pepper (Black)		Soya Bean Products
Pork		Squash
Tomato Products		Sugar
Sausage		Sweet Potatoes
Spices		Tapioca
Vegetable Gums*		Tea
Wheat		Vanilla Extract
Yeast		Water

Should you never eat a food if you are allergic to it?

The answer would depend upon how sensitive you are to the food. If every time you ate it, you had to be hospitalized, it would certainly be prudent not to eat that particular food. If, however, you find that wheat flour causes a slightly stuffy nose or a few hives, and you would like a cake for your birthday, there is certainly no reason why you cannot take an antihistamine and have a cake.

What is an unusually severe food allergy?

This type of allergy could be caused by the mere odour or slightest contact with a food. When someone cooks eggs, fish, or potatoes for example, it is possible to be in another room and know what is being cooked because you can smell the aroma in the air. These minute food particles (osmyls) in the air can cause allergy symptoms. Some persons are so allergic to nuts or fish that they cannot enter a cafeteria or walk past a counter in a store which contains these items. Some children are so sensitive to peanut butter that a jar cannot be opened in their home. It is possible for someone to eat eggs and cause allergies if he kisses someone who is sensitive to eggs because of the odour of eggs on his breath. This degree of sensitivity is fortunately rare. Patients who have an extreme sensitivity to eggs cannot use an egg shampoo because this will cause itching of the scalp or other symptoms of allergy.

Any patient who has such an extreme allergy to a food should wear a name tag stating that this is a problem (See page 261) and should carry emergency drugs at all times to be taken immediately whenever necessary.

What should a patient do if he ate a highly allergenic food?

Try to vomit. This will often happen immediately and is nature's way of helping. If it does not happen, a finger can be placed down the throat to cause vomiting. If a young child vomits, try to turn the child completely upside down so that nothing gets into his lungs.

If the patient cannot vomit, both an asthma drug and an antihistamine (See page 103) should be given immediately. The patient should be taken to the nearest physician or hospital, if there seems to be any obvious reason for concern. A drug which causes the bowels to move (aperient) should also be given if vomiting is not possible so that the offending food can be eliminated from the intestinal tract as quickly as possible.

Can someone die from eating a food to which he is extremely sensitive?

Yes. Fortunately such extreme allergy is rare but eating some foods (nuts, eggs, fish, or buckwheat) can cause this type of reaction. This sometimes happens if there is severe itching and swelling of the back of the tongue or the throat. Hoarseness or difficulty talking could indicate swelling near the upper wind pipe (trachea). Take an antihistamine and asthma drug immediately if these are available and rush to the nearest hospital.

There is hardly a food (or drug), however, which is not known, on occasion, to have caused a sudden immediate allergic reaction. Even a drop of milk has been known to cause a violent allergic response in some people.

If you eat a food to which you are allergic, when will symptoms occur?

An extreme allergy could cause an obvious reaction in seconds. Some foods may not cause difficulty for several hours. They may need to be thoroughly digested. A high blood level of digested food particles may be necessary before symptoms occur. Sometimes reactions to foods don't appear until a food has been eaten for several days or weeks. This can occur, for example, with a milk, wheat, or egg allergy.

A patient may not eat wheat for a few weeks and seem better. When he tries to eat wheat again, he may notice slight wheezing or that he consistently needs more drugs than before. The reappearance of symptoms can be so gradual that wheat is not suspected as being the cause of the allergy.

Although there are exceptions, fresh berries, fish, nuts (peanuts), and uncooked eggs tend to cause immediate allergic reactions. Cooked eggs, milk, corn, white potatoes, citrus fruits, chocolate, wheat, peas, and pork are more apt to cause reactions several hours after they are eaten.

The interval of time between eating a food and the appearance of symptoms can be altered by fatigue, emotions, exercise, or the way that a food was prepared. All these factors could affect digestion. One often finds, however, that a food which causes asthma repeatedly does this within a specific period of time which could vary from a few minutes in one individual or several hours in another person.

Could a person crave a food to which he is allergic?

Yes, this is often seen. It is frequently the food which is eaten in excess which causes difficulty. Children and adults sometimes have an unusual desire to eat the very food to which they are allergic. This is especially true for milk.

Do food allergies cause a natural aversion?

It is often possible to know the food to which an individual is allergic merely because the patient strongly dislikes or refuses to eat it. For example, a child who has to be forced or refuses to eat ice cream or chocolate, or to drink milk could have an allergy to milk or chocolate. Adults have similar dislikes which can be due to allergy.

A dislike of squash or liver would not cause suspicion concerning allergy because these foods are not particular favourites of many children or adults. Such a dislike could reflect a personal preference. It is not easy, especially in children, to tell an allergy from a preference. For this reason, very allergic children should *not* be forced to eat certain foods.

Does the amount or type of food affect an allergy?

Someone slightly sensitive to milk, might find that he could tolerate milk in cooked foods without difficulty, or possibly drink one glass a day, but if he attempted to drink 2 or 3 glasses a day, he would have symptoms.

The same could be true of eggs. Some people can eat eggs *only* in cooked foods. Raw, uncooked egg-white is much more likely to cause symptoms than a well-cooked hard boiled egg. Persons who cannot eat uncooked eggs would have difficulty drinking eggnogs or eating an egg-white frosting.

Can the season of the year affect food allergies?

It is possible to eat certain foods throughout most of the year and not have any symptoms. At a specific time, however, each year it may be noticed that these foods are temporarily no longer tolerated. Persons who have seasonal grass pollen problems may find that they cannot drink alcohol at that time. In Canada some patients can't eat melon or bananas during the weed pollen season.

Could a food allergy be related to a certain day of the week?

This is indeed possible. For example, it is not unusual for some Jewish families to eat lox (salmon) and bagels with cream cheese on Sunday morning. A person with a cheese or fish sensitivity could have symptoms every Sunday or early Monday. Many Italian families eat spaghetti or Armenian's eat lamb on a particular day each week. Catholics who eat fish or eggs on Friday can have allergies Friday night or Saturday. If someone's symptoms seem to occur regularly on a specific day each week, it could be related to a food which was eaten some time within a 12 to 24 hour period prior to the start of symptoms.

What should you do if the roof of your mouth itches?

This is a common complaint often noted after eating or drinking a food to which a person is allergic. An itchy mouth or throat and itchy ear canals can be noticed also during certain pollen seasons. When a patient has an itchy mouth, he should try to make an exact list of everything which has been placed in the mouth during the previous few hours (half day). The common belief that the same foods are eaten every day is seldom correct. A different brand of food, a new way of cooking it, an unfamiliar flavour, colouring, or spice can be the allergenic substance. Continually ask yourself: Why today and not yesterday? Why this evening and not this morning?

How long should you avoid a food which causes allergic symptoms?

If a food causes a severe alarming reaction, it should not be purposely eaten again at any time unless specifically advised and instructed by your physician. If at some time, however, a forbidden food is accidentally eaten, it probably can be eaten again *if* it caused no difficulty. Certain brands of a food can cause a severe reaction while another might not because of a different food additive or method of processing (See page 182). Allergies to eggs, nuts and fish often last a lifetime.

If food allergy symptoms are *not* alarming, it is possible to retest to see if the food allergy persists in approximately 6 to 18 months. For unexplained reasons, merely not eating a food for several months sometimes is followed by the disappearance of a mild food sensitivity. Sometimes a patient finds that a food allergy disappears for several months but later on the sensitivity recurs again. This food may have to be omitted from the diet again for several months before it can be tried again. Adult responses to foods often change with time. Fortunately infants with food allergy may completely outgrow this problem by the age of 1 or 2 years and the food allergy may never recur again.

Do patients with one food allergy, often have other food allergy?

Patients commonly have more than one food allergy. If a patient finds that his symptoms improve but are not eliminated when one food is not eaten, other foods should be checked. A clue to other possible offending foods can sometimes be provided by studying foods which cause symptoms in other members of a family.

Is skin testing for foods of value?

There is no uniform opinion. Physicians test by the method which is most familiar to them. European physicians believe that scratch food tests (See page 119) are very reliable.

Many physicians have little faith in food intradermal skin testing. There are often many positive reactions to foods by intradermal skin testing which are of no practical significance (See pages 117 to 122).

False allergy skin reactions can be due to difficulty in testing for digested or cooked foods. The protein portion of foods cause allergy. Cooking and digestion both alter proteins to such a degree that a test, for example, for raw egg-white on the arm or back might not reflect the response of the patient to a cooked digested egg.

Strongly positive skin test reactions to a food by either scratch or the intradermal testing can be valid. Dietary trials, however, are the final answer to any food test. When the patient eats the food, is he well or does it make him ill in some way? Regardless of the skin test reaction (scratch or intradermal), if the patient can eat the food without any difficulty, the food should not be denied to that patient.

Should skin tests be done for foods which cause serious reactions?

If you are certain that a food causes an alarming allergic reaction, there is no reason for a skin test. A test could possibly precipitate symptoms. It is sometimes necessary, however, to convince a mother not repeatedly to try to feed some food to her child.

Scratch skin testing is a relatively safe method to help demonstrate to all concerned that a particular food can cause an allergic reaction.

Do special injection treatments help food allergies?

This type of therapy is not effective. A child who is acutely allergic to eggs is not desensitized with a series of injections. This is potentially very hazardous procedure. If the child will refrain from eating eggs in any form, including in cakes for example, the egg allergy may be outgrown. Under these circumstances, few will retain their egg allergy through to adult life. Food allergies at any age are socially a nuisance, but only a very few allergists would undertake treating food allergy by injection treatment.

One school of allergists claim success in using a provocation and neutralizing injection method for diagnosing and treating food allergies. They believe that the use of drops of food under the tongue is helpful. Some allergists strongly doubt these claims and scientific attempts are presently being made to prove or deny them.

HOW AND WHEN SHOULD YOU CHECK FOR A FOOD ALLERGY?

What is the most reliable way to detect a food allergy?

A diet is the most accurate method to check for food allergy. There are two distinct parts. The first is *omission* of a food or foods to determine if this helps the allergy. The second part is to *re-add* these same foods to the diet to see if this causes a recurrence of the allergy. Medical research may eventually make it possible to diagnose food allergies reliably by a blood examination but this is not possible at the present time. A better method of food allergy detection is constantly being sought but we have no single widely accepted and readily available test other than diets.

What overlooked clue helps greatly in food allergy detection?

If a patient has NO allergy symptoms at some time, keep an EXACT record of everything which was eaten during this period. These foods cannot be major causes of this patient's allergies. This list can be used as a beginning diet to which new single foods can be added every few days to help determine which foods are causing symptoms. For example, if you feel wonderful on a particular day and are still fine the next morning, the foods you ate the previous day were alright. When you are not well if you eat these same identical foods, your diet will not contain any major allergenic food to further complicate your allergy.

Do you need a physician's help to do dietary studies?

Many individuals are on diets for multiple reasons without supervision by a physician. If a person is beyond the infant age and in relatively good health, a two-week diet should not be harmful. Diets, however, need a physician's supervision if they last longer than 2 weeks or are being carried out in an infant. In some patients omitting a food may cause dramatic improvement in just a day or two, in others improvement may not occur for one or more weeks. Although many allergic food problems can be detected using a 2 week diet, others will be missed.

Are dietary trials difficult?

Dietary trials can be *extremely* difficult and require determination. If an individual is not willing to read the labels on *all* food containers, errors will be made. *Every* possible source of the slightest amount of the food which is to be omitted must be eliminated or problems will arise and an incorrect interpretation made. For example, if an adult is allergic to milk, he is *not* on a milk-free diet if he is receiving skim milk, pudding, cottage cheese, baked goods, butter, many types of bread, or any item which contains the smallest quantity of milk (See page 183).

Diets often create tension within a family. Youngsters do not understand why they cannot eat what they want and have always eaten. Parents feel guilty denying their children foods they should eat. Other children or adults in a family may give an allergic child a little bit of the forbidden food because they feel sorry for him. This greatly delays or makes the determination of exactly what is causing an allergy impossible. If a child needs a diet, it often helps if the entire family can be placed on the diet.

Do not attempt dietary trials unless you are truly determined to carry the diet through to completion. All too often a patient begins a diet in a half-hearted manner and repeatedly forgets and eats a small quantity of the foods which are not to be eaten. After weeks of dieting, no conclusions can be made because of innumerable errors. How much better to have done the diet correctly *once* for a 2 week period and to know for sure if foods are a factor or not.

When should dietary trials be avoided?

1.   Foods should never be re-added to a diet if the patient has an infection. It would be difficult to determine whether the addition of the food or the infection were causing any flare of allergy. You can omit or not eat certain foods during infection but never add them back at that

time. If infection seems to be passing among different members of the family, re-add foods after that problem has subsided.

    2.   Do not carry out diets at a time of the year when pollens and moulds spores are in the air (See page 166). If you re-added a food on a high pollen count day and then had symptoms, it would be difficult to tell what caused the problem.

    3.   Food studies should be delayed if a patient had had recent surgery or a severely traumatic life crisis.

    4.   Dietary studies would be indicated only if a person's history suggested food allergy could be a problem (See page 158).

    5.   If a patient is underweight and poorly nourished, attempt no dietary manipulation without a doctor's supervision.

    6.   If there is a violent allergy to a food, no attempt to study the effects of this food can be considered without a specialist's advice. (See page 5).

    7.   Dietary testing should be avoided if the patient is eating in restaurants, travelling, camping, or on a holiday. At these times it would be too difficult to control exactly what was being eaten.

    8.   Dietary studies should be timed so they will not cause problems during family birthdays or celebrations.

Why are diets hard to interpret?

The results of dietary studies are often clear-cut and definite. A person stops eating a food and seems better; the food is re-added and the patient is worse. If this repeatedly happens, there is little doubt that the food is at fault. In some patients, however, when a food is omitted, the individual seems a little but not completely better. Other factors such as dust, pets, or other foods may be continuing to cause symptoms of allergies. When a suspected allergenic food is eaten again, the patient seems to be a bit worse, but again the change is not dramatic. This is one reason why a contrast helps when doing a food allergy study. The food initially must be omitted *in all forms*, and later on *eaten in excess* when it is re-added to the diet.

Which special problems hinder diet study interpretation?

As previously mentioned, eating the "wrong" foods (See page 169) and the presence of pollen (See page 166) can make diets difficult to interpret

The need for antihistamines or asthma drugs can complicate diet study. For example, if someone is using three antihistamines a day to relieve his symptoms and continues to need three antihistamines a day when he's on the diet, this would indicate that he had not improved. If, however, he found that during the diet he needed no medicine or only one antihistamine a day, this might indicate that omitting a food helped the allergies. When the offending food is re-added in excess, if the symptoms are poorly controlled on four antihistamines a day, this would confirm that an offending food probably has been found. See Table 12-31 b c.

Evaluation of diets is frequently made difficult because of exposure to another allergenic substance. For example, suppose someone thought he was allergic to chocolate because he seemed to improve when he stopped eating it. The day chocolate is re-added to his diet, however, he decides to clean a dusty basement and nose symptoms are noticed. He could interpret that the chocolate caused the symptoms, when the cause could have been the dusty basement. For this reason, repeat any dietary challenge which causes symptoms because it could be a coincidence and not a cause and effect relationship.

One last factor often clouds decisions about food allergy. It can be exemplified by the patient who is possibly allergic to wheat. When wheat is eliminated, he is better. When it is re-added, he is worse. If is difficult, however, to eat normally if one cannot eat foods containing wheat. The tendency, therefore, is to attribute the recurrence of symptoms not to wheat, but to visiting a friend or being near a dog. Psychologically, it is easier to accept not being near a dog than it is to stop eating wheat. A person who has allergies must face facts squarely. Pretending won't make the allergies go away.

How can you be certain that a food does *not* cause an allergy?

If a patient remains the same when a food is eliminated from his diet and when it is eaten in excess, it means he is probably not allergic to that food. There would be no need to repeat the dietary trial.

If a person's allergies seem slightly worse when a food is first re-added, but *while continuing to eat that food* he seems to feel better, the food in question is *not* a factor causing allergy. For example, suppose you have not eaten eggs for 2 weeks. The first day when you re-add eggs to your diet, you eat 4. Your nose and chest seem worse. The next day you eat 4 eggs again and seem alright. You continue to eat 4 eggs a day and stay well. This means that eggs cannot be causing your allergy even though you seemed somewhat worse the first day. Something else caused you to have symptoms at that time. If you had been truly allergic to eggs and you continued to eat 4 eggs each day, your symptoms should have become more and more evident as every day passed. As soon as you noticed that you felt progressively worse, you should have stopped eating that food.

When adding foods to a diet, what is "an excess"?

Adding a food "in excess" to your diet means eating or drinking more than normal. If you normally eat 2 eggs a day, 4 is an excess. If you normally drink 1 glass of milk a day, 2 is an excess.

HOW CAN YOU DO AN
ALLERGY DIETARY TRIAL?

What are the major types of food allergy diets?
There are 4 basic dietary methods to detecting food allergies:
1. *Single Food Elimination Diet* (when you suspect one food)
2. *A "Good" and "Bad" Day Food Diary* (when your symptoms don't occur every day)
3. *Provocation Diet* (when your symptoms aren't severe—and you don't want to diet)
4. *Multiple Food Allergy Diet* (when you have daily symptoms but suspect no particular food.)

1. *Single Food Elimination Diet:*
This type of diet would be indicated if a person were allergic to only 1 or 2 foods (See page 167). Some single foods which often cause allergies are: milk, eggs, wheat, fish, peanuts, chocolate, tomatoes, white potatoes, or citrus fruits.
Eliminate the food in question from the diet *in every form in which it exists* (See page 169). If the food is causing allergies, improvement should be obvious in a day or 2 or within the 2 week period. After 2 weeks *or* as soon as you notice the diet has eliminated your symptoms, the food in question should be re-added to your diet in gradually increasing amounts. If you find that you can re-add the food and eat as much as you like for 3 to 7 days without difficulty, it is unlikely that the tested food is the cause of your problem. (Re-add most foods for 3 days, but re-add milk, wheat, or eggs for a full week.) If the addition of the food causes no apparent difficulty, there is no need to check this food again. It is probably not related to your allergies.
If, however, when a food is eliminated your symptoms disappear and when you re-add it to your diet your symptoms recur, it is suggestive that the suspected food is causing difficulty. To be certain, however, that the cause and effect relationship exists, it is best if this Single Food Elimination Diet is repeated 2 or 3 times to prove that the food in question really is the cause of the difficulty.

2. *A "Good" and "Bad" Day Food Diary:*
This is a relatively easy way to find out if a food causes *infrequent* symptoms. In other words, the patient is fine most of the time, and then suddenly becomes very ill.
The food diary is helpful in detecting the cause of a wide range of symptoms such as wheezing, welts, or skin rashes, nose allergies, joint pains, digestive upsets, and behaviour or disposition problems. If a person is entirely well on a particular day and the next morning he continues

to feel fine, it means that during the previous 24 hours, he probably has not eaten any foods to which he is allergic. The list should contain every item placed in the mouth during that 24-hour period. This includes drugs, toothpaste, mouthwash. This list should be called the "good" day list. At least 5 such "good" days should be recorded.

If a patient who has been fine, suddenly has some allergic symptom on a particular day, this is called a "bad" day. All food items eaten or medicines taken during the previous, waking, 12-hour period should be recorded. If the undesirable symptoms appear upon awakening in the morning, it could be due to something which was eaten late in the after-noon or evening of the previous day. If the symptom, however, appeared in the evening hours, it quite possibly is something that was eaten on that same day. Once again, records should be kept for several "bad" days.

By comparing foods eaten on these "good" and "bad" days, it should be possible to detect certain ones which were eaten *only* on "bad" days, not on the "'good" days. These foods can be checked individually by omitting them from the diet for approximately a week and then feeding each in excess to see if one produces allergic symptoms.

One must be cautioned to keep very explicit records. It is not adequate merely to list ice cream, but one should state what brand and flavour of ice cream. One extra ingredient (dye, spice, or flavouring) in a certain brand could be the cause of someone's problem.

Such lists are extremely helpful whenever a patient has severe aller-gies. If you know that certain foods can be eaten without difficulty, you can eat these anytime, especially when your allergies are a problem. This way you can be sure that what you eat is not making your allergy worse.

Example: (abbreviated form)

"Good" Day	*"Bad" Day*	*Foods to Check*
X Bread X	X Bread X	
X Milk X	X Milk X	
Carrots*	Peanut Butter	Peanut Butter
Orange Juice*	Grape Jelly	Grape Jelly
Broccoli*	Spinach	Spinach
X Beef X	X Beef X	

*These foods cannot be causing symptoms because no difficulty oc-curred on the day that these were eaten. "Crossed" foods cannot be a problem because these caused no difficulty on the "good" day.

3. *Provocation Diet:*

This diet is the easiest because no elimination of any food is required. When doing this diet the patient has to eat an excessive amount of the food which might be causing allergic symptoms for a week. Obviously this type of challenge could cause severe allergic reactions so it should be done *cautiously* with your physician's help unless your allergic problems are not extreme. If a patient remains well when an excess of a certain food is eaten, it is most unlikely that the tested food is causing allergy. If he progressively becomes more and more ill, however, the food in question is *probably* a factor related to his allergies.

Caution in interpretation is needed. For example, a patient may be well and then become very ill 2 days after the suspected food has been added to the diet. It is possible that the patient came in contact with some other allergenic substance on that particular day. For this reason, the food which is being checked should be eliminated from the diet. When the patient is again well, that particular food item can be re-added to see if it causes difficulties again. If the food repeatedly causes allergies, it must be omitted from the diet for at least several months.

4. *Multiple Food Allergy Diet:*

This diet often solves the allergy problem but it is by far the most difficult for both the allergic person and the rest of his family. The patient can eat only a few foods which seldom cause allergy. This dietary method is often necessary when the previous methods have failed to reveal the offending allergic foods. If this diet, however, is tried for 14 days and the patient does not improve and when he suddenly eats a regular diet he is not worse, it suggests that a food allergy is not present. This, however, assumes that there was rigid adherence to the diet, that there was no food in the Multiple Food Allergy Diet to which the patient was allergic and that the diet was carried out for an adequate length of time.

If a person is allergic to several foods, a diet is allowed which includes fruits and certain types of meat and vegetables. The foods which cannot be eaten include wheat, milk, eggs, nuts, chocolate, fish, and major corn products. It is very difficult to plan appetizing meals while omitting these common foods. To make it easier, lists of various food items which *can be* eaten, with recipes for common food combinations have been outlined on page 178. If an individual prefers certain meats or beverages, for example, he can select whatever he favours most from any of the lists. Absolutely nothing, however, can be added to the diet or substituted for any item unless it is definitely listed. The selected diet, of course, should not include any food to which an individual is obviously sensitive. In general, the diet should be followed only by individuals who are over 1½ years of age and should not be attempted for a period longer than 2 weeks. While many allergists do longer dietary studies, this is certainly not advisable unless you are so advised by your physician.

For a week or so before and during the period of time when the diet is being carried out, careful daily records should be made concerning each of a patient's symptoms. The amount of medication which is necessary each day should be listed (See Table 2 page 176). By studying these records, it is often *much easier* to decide if the diet was helpful or not. If a person's symptoms and need for medicine remained the same before and during the diet, it would indicate that the diet was not helpful. After the 14-day diet, that individual should not only resume his ordinary diet, but should be urged to eat an excessive amount of wheat, milk, eggs, nuts (peanut butter), chocolate, fish, or major corn products (whole kernel corn or popcorn). An individual who does not seem better in any way when he is on the diet, and is not worse in any way when the specified foods are re-added in excess, is probably not allergic to the foods which were investigated. (See page 174).

TABLE 1

RECORDS TO DETECT FOOD ALLERGY

Code
0 = no symptoms or trouble
1 = slight symptoms
3 = severe symptoms
2 = anything between slight
    and severe
X = date FOOD was added

The following records in an abbreviated form show how you can tell if a certain food causes allergies or not. Records should be kept for several days before the diet is started and for the entire period during which foods are being added. Such records make it much easier to form conclusions about a diet.

SAMPLE RECORD SHOWING FOOD ALLERGY

Symptoms	day	1 2 3 4 5	6 7 8 9 10	11 12 13	
nose allergies		1 0 1 2 1	2 3 3 3 3	2 1 1	
eye allergies		0 0 1 0 0	1 1 1 2 2	1 0 0	conclusion:
chest allergies		2 1 2 2 1	2 3 3 3 3	3 2 2	food causes nose,
skin allergies		1 0 1 0 0	1 2 2 2 2	1 1 1	eye, chest, skin
disposition (irritable)		1 0 1 1 0	1 2 3 3 3	2 1 1	and disposition
infection		0 0 0 0 0	0 0 0 0 0	0 0 0	changes.

Drugs (number used each day)

for nose, eyes, or skin	1 0 2 2 1	2 3 3 3 3	2 2 1	Symptoms and
for asthma or cough	2 1 2 2 1	3 4 4 4 4	3 2 2	need for drugs

Food added (days 6 to 10)   XXXXX
(Food omitted from days
1 to 5 and after day 10)

increased after
food was added.

TABLE 2.

RECORDS TO DETECT FOOD ALLERGY

Code
0 = no symptoms or trouble
1 = slight symptoms
3 = severe symptoms
2 = anything between slight
and severe
X = date FOOD was added

The following records in an abbreviated form show how you can tell if a certain food causes allergies or not. Records should be kept for several days before the diet is started and for the entire period during which foods are being added. Such records make it much easier to form conclusions about a diet.

SAMPLE RECORD SHOWING NO FOOD ALLERGY

Symptoms	day	1 2 3 4 5	6 7 8 9 10	11 12 13	
nose allergies		1 0 1 2 1	1 0 2 0 1	1 2 0	
eye allergies		0 0 1 0 0	1 0 1 1 0	0 1 0	
chest allergies		2 1 2 2 1	2 2 1 2 2	1 1 2	
skin allergies		1 0 1 0 0	1 1 0 0 0	1 1 1	conclusion:
disposition (irritable)		1 0 1 1 0	1 1 1 0 1	1 0 0	food does not
infection		0 0 0 0 0	0 0 0 0 0	0 0 0	cause allergy

Drugs (number used each day)

for nose, eyes, or skin	1 0 2 2 1	2 1 1 1 2	0 1 1	
for asthma or cough	2 1 2 2 1	2 2 1 1 2	1 2 2	

Food added (6 to 10)   **X X X X X**   Symptoms were
  (Food omitted from days   about the same
  1 to 5 and after day 10)   before and after
                                                                              food; so were
                                                                              drugs.

If, however, a patient seemed to be markedly improved (fewer symptoms and need for less medicine) (See page 170) during the time when the highly allergic foods were omitted from his diet, it would indicate that any of these foods could be causing symptoms. The patient would, therefore, have to be placed on the same diet for another 2 weeks. One at a time, the following foods would be added to the diet for a week to determine which one caused the reappearance of allergic symptoms: milk, wheat, eggs, nuts, chocolate, fish or major corn products. Once the patient has determined which food is causing difficulty, it should be omitted in all forms from his diet for a period of 6 to 18 months. If milk and soya milk are omitted from a growing child's diet, calcium is needed for normal bone growth. (See page 184).

When would the Multiple Food Allergy Diet *not* be helpful?
This diet would not help any individual who was allergic to corn (in trace amounts), citrus fruits, tomatoes, white potatoes, chicken, cinnamon, and to various food flavourings, dyes, and food additives. These foods might have to be individually checked (See page 174) if there was a suspicion concerning one of them. Some types of food allergies are difficult to diagnose. A person with many food allergies probably could not determine the offending foods without the help of a well-trained specialist.

Is the problem solved once you find the allergy causing food?
No, unfortunately this is only the beginning. It is extremely difficult consistently to avoid some foods. Eating in restaurants or schools will often expose a patient to a food in a hidden form. Many people would rather eat the food and have symptoms, than be inconvenienced by continually trying to detect where this food might happen to be found.

The problem of making a diet palatable and enticing is often a major challenge if a patient is allergic to a food which normally is a major part of his diet. Parties at home or at school, adult social events, or obligations related to employment can create a crisis emotionally or physically. There is no easy answer. Living with a major food allergy requires an unusual amount of maturity.

The treatment should never be worse than the disease. If eating a certain food causes slight symptoms which are easily controlled by medicine and have no immediate or future bad effect on your health, by all means eat it. Such decisions, however, should be discussed with your physician because non-medically trained persons often make incorrect decisions concerning what is or is not harmful to their health.

Do you always have to check for a food allergy?
No. Some children and adults don't like certain foods and have no desire to try to eat them. If you never eat fish and do not want to eat fish, you do not have to eat it. Merely try to remember, however, that if and when you do decide to eat a little fish, you should try to notice if that food causes any ill effects which could be allergic.

MULTIPLE FOOD ALLERGY DIET

This diet omits all milk and dairy products, wheat (bread, cake, baked goods), eggs, nuts, chocolate, fish, and major corn products. It allows meat, fruits, and vegetables. *Only* the following foods can be selected, combined, and eaten in any quantity for *any* meal. *No* other food items can be eaten or used in preparation or cooking. If an item is not listed, it should *NOT* be eaten. If one of the suggested foods causes obvious or suspected allergy, do not include it in *your* individual diet.

Beverages

Soya bean Milk
Juice or carbonated beverages:
    Orange   Apple
    Grapefruit Peach
    Lemon   Pineapple
    Grape   Pear
    Cranberry
Coffee Rich
Tea
Coffee, black only
Liquid gelatin

Cereals or Grains

Oatmeal
Barley
Rice:
    Flour
    Spanish
Ry-Krisp, non-seasoned

Meat

Bacon
Beef:
    Pot Roast
    Stew
    Swiss Steak
Chicken:
    Baked
    Salad
Pork:
    Chops
    Roast
Ham
Liver
Kosher all-meat
    Weiners and
    Bologna
Hash
Meatloaf

Fruits

Bananas
Apple:
    Raw
    Baked
    Sauce
Grapes:
    Raisins
    Jelly
Peaches
Pears
Oranges
Grapefruit
Tangerine
Pineapple
Fruit Cocktail

Miscellaneous

Egg-free Baking
    Powder (obtain
    at Health Food
    Store)
Molasses
Water
Vegetable (not
    corn) Cooking Oil
Kosher Margarine
Mayonnaise
Potato Starch
Potato Flour
Potato Meal
Bacon Drippings

Vegetables

		Desserts
Cabbage:	Brussel Sprouts	Gelatin:
Cole Slaw	Baked Squash	Orange
Carrots	Chives	Lemon
White Potato:	Tossed Salad with	Cherry
Mashed	French Dressing	Brown Sugar Bars
Fried		Apple Crisp
Boiled		Cherry Crisp
Baked		Gingerbread
French Fries		Soya bean Milk Ice
Chips		Cream
Salad		Tapioca
Flour		(Use gelatin mould for cake)
Sweet Potato:		
Baked		*Condiments*
Candied		
Green Beans		Salt
Tomatoes:		Pepper
Raw		Sugar
Canned		White
Lettuce		Brown
Spinach		Ginger
Celery		Cinnamon
Green Pepper		Vinegar
Broccoli		White
Cucumbers		Cider
Beets		Paprika
Asparagus		Bayleaf
Onions		Thyme

What is a fast way to determine if a food is causing some allergy?

There is one quick way to detect a food allergy, but it is not a particularly easy way and would be advisable only in older children and adults. Many persons have symptoms such as nausea, nose allergies, headaches, or asthma every single day for years. You can often detect if it is a food causing the problem by not eating for 24 hours. Drink only distilled water or possibly spring water. Try to eat nothing. If you become shaky, you may take some honey. This rarely causes allergy. If the medical problem disappears for the first time in a long time, it means that, for certain, a food is the cause of your problem. Be sure to stop mouthwash and toothpaste at the same time and take no medicines or drugs unless they are absolutely essential. Your physician can help slowly to guide you back to a normal diet, and help you find the offending food items as you eat more and more foods.

If your medical problem remains entirely unchanged after a 24-hour fast, it is unlikely that a food is at fault.

Can you prevent a food allergy reaction?

The only way to be certain, is to avoid eating the food causing trouble. There is some indication in children that immediate symptoms caused by foods can be prevented by swallowing (not inhaling) disodium cromoglycate *before* the food is eaten.

Do vitamins cause or help allergies?

Cod liver capsules can cause difficulty in fish allergic patients. Vitamin D and thiamine (B_1) have sometimes been said to cause allergic problems. Vitamin allergies, however, are rarely noted or diagnosed. Problems could be due to the vitamin, dye, flavouring, or binder used in the vitamin preparation.

There are some claims that vitamins, especially C and various types of B such as pantothenic acid will help eliminate allergic problems. To date there are no scientific clearly substantiated studies in humans to verify these claims.

How can you detect a vitamin allergy?

You can try to determine if a vitamin is causing minor allergy symptoms. The first step would be to see if a different coloured vitamin of approximately the same composition caused the same symptoms. If a change in the colour of the tablet eliminated the problem, it would indicate that a dye might be at fault.

If the vitamin which you have been using contains many vitamins, attempt to secure a few vitamin tablets which contain a single vitamin of each type. By trying one at a time, you should be able to determine exactly which one is at fault. Vitamin B_1 is also called thiamine hydrochloride; B_2 is riboflavin; and C is ascorbic acid.

If the above investigation does not reveal the cause of the difficulty, check with your doctor.

SPECIAL FOOD PROBLEMS

Are food labels accurate?

Not always. Labels can be correct, incomplete, deceptive, or inaccurate. For example, a product which contains milk may only state that it contains sodium caseinate, which is a milk product. It is also possible for some items labelled "milk-free" to contain a small amount of milk. Because the milk content is small, labels can sometimes say that they do not contain milk. In most patients this would not be a problem, but in others the smallest amount could cause symptoms.

Another common example is related to eggs. The label may not say an item contains eggs, but instead will say vitellin, ovovitellin, livetin, ovomucoid, ovomucin, albumin, or globulin. Egg yolk can be called lecithin. All are egg proteins and could cause allergies (See page 184).

Do similar foods cause allergy?

Certain similar foods *often* cause allergies. A person allergic to one might be allergic to others in each group. Examples are:

Coffee – Tea – Cola – Caffeine – containing medicines
Sage – Mint – Peppermint
Carrot – Celery – Cumin – Coreander
Egg – Chicken – Turkey
Peas – Peanuts – Licorice – Possibly Certain Beans – Soya bean
Lobster – Crab – Shrimp

In these groups, a person may or may not be allergic to the others:

Orange – Lemon – Lime – Grapefruit – Tangerine – Kumquat (Citric acid is alright)
Wheat – Oats – Rye – Barley – Rice

Do food additives cause allergies?

There is an ever increasing variety of substances presently added to innumerable food items. Common additives are:

1. Preservatives – to prevent spoilage (calcium propionate)
2. Antioxidants – to prevent or retard rancidity – butylated hydroxytoluene
3. Sequestrants – to bind up trace elements of metals and make them inactive, such as sodium citrate in soft drinks.
4. Surfactants – to help liquids which might tend to separate to combine into a stable mixture. These include lecithin and monoglycerides.
5. Thickeners or stabilizers – to improve consistency (pectin, tragacanth, or acacia).
6. Bleaching and maturing agents – such as chlorine
7. Buffers, acids and alkalies – to modify taste
8. Citric acid to intensify fruit flavour, or sodium carbonate to decrease acidity in canned vegetables
9. Non-nutritive sweeteners
10. Nutrient supplements – for example, iron, thiamine, and riboflavin
11. Pesticides
12. Flavouring agents – mono-sodium glutamate (Chinese foods containing this sometimes cause headaches)

13. Salicyclates

One or more of the above could be found in butter, processed cheese, ice cream, bread, cake, cake mixes, breakfast cereals, peanut butter, salad or cooking oils, processed meats, various beverages, beer, jams or jellies, gelatin desserts, and cookies or crackers.

Claims regarding the safety and hazards of these various additives are being studied to determine their effect in humans. In the meantime, efforts should be made to urge proper labelling of all foods so that sensitive persons can more effectively avoid chemical additives.

Which artificial food colours are most apt to cause allergies?

There are many acceptable azo dyes to colour foods and drugs. The red dye amaranth commonly causes symptoms. It is in red or purple coloured medicines, candies, and gelatin. The other dye frequently causing allergies is yellow tartrazine. This dye is found in yellow or orange margarine, medicines, coating on pills, some vegetables or fruits, and gelatin. Aspirin sensitive patients frequently also have a reaction to products containing tartrazine.

Should egg-allergic patients avoid eating *female* chicken?

As strange as it may seem, some egg-allergic patients cannot eat *female* chicken, but have no difficulty when they eat a *capon, rooster,* or *male chicken.* This cannot readily be explained. If you are allergic to eggs and can eat any type of chicken, do not be concerned. If you find, however, that chicken sometimes causes symptoms, you should determine the sex of the chicken which you eat.

Are there special milks which seldom cause allergy?

It is possible to buy heat denatured milks. This means the milk proteins which cause allergies have been altered markedly by heating during the processing of the milk. The modification of various milk preparations differs but the proteins may be altered so much that a patient who can't drink regular milk might be able to tolerate altered milk products. Your physician can best advise you concerning the various types which are available.

Should milk sensitive individuals avoid beef?

Milk allergic patients can eat beef, but each person must be considered individually. If you find your allergy symptoms recur when you eat beef or drink milk, both items should be avoided. Papain contamination of beef can cause symptoms. (See page 188).

Will adults or older children drink soya bean milk?

Many will not. It should be mixed as directed on the container and chilled. Some will take soya bean milk on cereal, but will not drink it. It is more tasty if a teaspoon of vanilla and sugar is added to each can and it is whipped with a blender. Soya bean milk can cause bowel movements to become more soft than normal.

Is there a soya bean milk ice cream?

Yes, this can be made very simply in the following manner:

MECHANICAL FREEZER METHOD

4 – 13-oz. cans soya bean milk concentrate (do not dilute with water).
2 – packets (1 tablespoon/packet) unflavoured gelatin. Soften in ½ cup cold water.
1 – cup sugar. Add to the gelatin and heat slowly to dissolve sugar and gelatin; cool.
½ – cup clear corn syrup.
¼ – cup salad/cooking oil.
2 – tablespoons plus 1 teaspoon vanilla extract.
Mix all ingredients and freeze in one-gallon or five-quart ice cream freezer. After the mix is frozen, it may be stored in an electric freezer but it can become more icy.
The vanilla flavoured soya bean ice cream is better if berries, peaches, bananas, pineapple or oranges are added to it. Mash or purée the fruit in a blender, depending upon your individual tastes and allergies prior to use.

Is it possible to avoid all milk products?

It is not easy. Milk is found in many items. Beverages to replace milk include dark tea or black coffee, juices, carbonated beverages or soya bean milk. Children like to drink warm dilute liquid gelatin or put it on their cereal.

Recipe books for soya bean milk use are available. Soya bean milk cannot be used by persons allergic to soya beans or possibly peanuts or peas.

A person on a milk-free diet should *not* drink skimmed milk or other types of cow's or goat's milk. A list of foods commonly containing milk is on page 180. Milk chocolate contains milk.

If milk cannot be taken, how can calcium be supplied?

Growing children who cannot drink milk can obtain sufficient calcium to provide normal bone growth if they eat other dairy products such as cheese, or drink a milk substitute such as soya bean milk. If a patient has such a severe milk allergy that no milk can be taken in any form, calcium must be provided from other sources. Some children cannot or will not drink soya bean milk. Calcium also can be provided by feeding foods which are high in calcium, providing these do not cause allergy. Other sources are calcium gluconate or calcium lactate tablets or liquid. These can cause a digestive upset and diarrhoea in some patients.

How much calcium does a person need?

The daily requirement for calcium gradually rises through childhood until girls are about 16 and boys 18 years of age. Infants under one year require 400 to 600 mg per day. Children aged 1 year to 12 years require 700 to 1200 mg per day. Children from 12 to 18 years of age require about 1200 to 1400 mg per day. Adults from about age 18 to 75 years require about 800 mg per day.

What is the calcium content in some common foods?

1 cup milk provides 288 mg. Calcium
1 oz. (30 gm) salmon with bones provides 51 mg. Calcium
1 oz. (30 gm) sardines provides 115 mg. Calcium
1 oz. (30 gm) shrimp provides 35 mg. Calcium
½ cup (90 gm) beans, dry (cooked or canned) provides 45 mg.
½ cup lima beans provides 42 mg. Calcium
2/3 cup (100 gm) parsnips provides 45 mg. Calcium
1 oz. (30 gm) cheddar cheese provides 218 mg. Calcium
1 oz. cheese spread or foods provides 160 mg. Calcium
¼ cup cottage cheese provides 53 mg. Calcium
1 cup soya bean milk provides about 200 mg. Calcium

Do any clues help to pinpoint fish or egg allergy?

In relation to observing religious fasts, it is possible to eat foods which cause allergies. For example, allergic symptoms commonly occur in Catholics late Friday and Saturday morning because fish or eggs are eaten to replace meat. Sometimes the allergic person does not actually eat fish, but has symptoms if fish is brought into the home. Each weekend he becomes ill because he can smell the odour of fish eaten by others.

How can eggs be avoided?

Aside from being careful to avoid eggs in their usual form, one must be careful to avoid an eggnog or egg-white containing frostings. Many forms of candy or sweets contain eggs. Most baked goods contain eggs. (See page 181 re lecithin). It is possible to bake without using eggs if one uses an egg-free baking powder. (Obtainable at health food stores.) For each egg omitted from a recipe, an extra half teaspoon of egg-free baking powder is added. For example, if a recipe requires 2 eggs and 1 teaspoon of baking powder, the egg allergic person would omit the egg but use 2 teaspoons of egg-free baking powder. A list of common egg-containing foods is on page 184.

Which fish cause allergy?

There are many types of fish. Some persons are allergic to tuna, salmon, or trout. If a patient cannot eat tuna, he might very well also have difficulty with salmon or trout. Other patients cannot eat other fish such as cod, halibut, haddock, sole, pike, perch, and white fish. If someone could not eat one of these, he could conceivably have trouble from the others. Similarly, persons sensitive to one crustacean (clam, lobster, and shrimp), or to one mollusc (clams, oysters, and scallops) can have symptoms from any of the others (See page 181).

What special precautions should be advised regarding fish allergy?

Many fish sensitive patients, in addition to not being able to eat fish, cannot tolerate touching or the odour of fish. This can cause difficulty, for example, in cafeterias or restaurants, at work or school where fish is served, or in meat markets or stores where fish might be sold. Fishing could cause symptoms. Cleaning fish tanks or feeding fish in tanks can produce symptoms. Some persons are sensitive to some ingredients in fish food (i.e. flaxseed). Pizza, clam chowder, or fish soups, and party dips can cause trouble. Patients allergic to fish should never take cod liver oil tablets or capsules.

Caramel or tan-coloured glue is often made from fish. Licking envelopes, stamps, stickers, picture hangers, or stamp collections can cause symptoms. Books, boxes or even furniture which are glued together, especially when they are old, can be a problem.

White paste is seldom allergenic. Clear, colourless glues, such as the type used to cement model toys, have strong odours and can cause difficulty which is unrelated to a fish allergy.

Do combinations of foods ever cause allergies?

Occasional patients find they can eat a food without difficulty, but whenever this food is combined with another certain food, symptoms of allergy occur. For example, some patients can eat shrimp or they can drink alcoholic beverages. Either alone would cause no difficulty. If, however, shrimp are eaten at the same time that the alcoholic beverage is consumed, it causes definite allergic symptoms. Another similar food combination is prunes and beer.

Combination food allergies are much more difficult to detect than single food problems. Patients who keep records of everything eaten before every sudden allergic episode may be able to detect combination foods which are causing symptoms.

What can someone substitute for bread?

Various bread substitutes are available as well as many recipes for baking bread which does not contain wheat. Many of these breads, however, are hard and coarse. Their taste is so unlike regular bread that many patients refuse to eat them. It should be remembered that most types of bread (potato, rice, rye) contain wheat flour. It is possible to purchase rice, rye, or potato flour from health stores but it is difficult to bake a tasty bread without the use of wheat flour.

Is it possible to make gravy without wheat flour?

A thickening agent such as arrowroot, corn starch, or potato starch can be used providing these items do not cause allergic symptoms.

Which types of corn cause allergies?

Corn is an important grain used frequently in some parts of the world and it commonly causes allergy. It is found in many products listed on page 163. It is used in the preparation of both Bourbon whisky and beer. Patients who are corn allergic can have difficulty from intravenous fluids in a hospital because these can contain dextrose or corn sugar. It is possible to be sensitive to corn syrup, but not to have difficulty with whole kernel corn or pop corn. Most soya bean milks contain corn.

Are allergies to cinnamon common?

Cinnamon is possibly the most common spice causing allergies. It is used in a variety of sweetened foods such as cakes, chili, candies, cookies, ketchup, prepared meats, apple dishes and chewing gum. Patients who are allergic to this spice may also have difficulty from bay leaf and some toothpaste or mouthwash.

Is there a substitute for chocolate?

There is a form of chocolate made from soya beans which can be purchased in health food or grocery stores. It has the appearance and aroma of chocolate, but the taste is different.

White or coloured chocolate is as allergenic as brown chocolate. Milk chocolate contains milk and chocolate. If chocolate is to be tested as a cause of allergy during a period of time when milk *cannot* be taken, the patient should try only dark chocolate, cocoa, and cola beverages.

Where are citrus fruits found?

The citrus family includes oranges, grapefruits, lemons, limes, tangerines, and kumquats. A patient may be allergic to one, several, or all of these. If someone is allergic to citrus, he might have to avoid juices, soda pop, gelatin, hard candy, medicines, cough drops, or any other item containing citrus fruit flavour. Surprisingly citric acid may not cause symptoms.

Why are nut allergies perplexing?

Nut allergy tends to be a very individual problem. Some persons are slightly or extremely allergic to only one type of nut, others to many or all types. Persons who are very sensitive can react violently or even die from the taste of a nut. The odour of the nut, or a speck of almond or walnut extract flavouring in baked goods, cake icing, chocolate or a carbonated beverage can cause extreme symptoms. Nut allergic patients may or may not be allergic to peanuts.

Peanuts are not nuts, but legumes or in the pea family. Persons with peanut allergy can be so allergic that the smell from an open peanut butter jar can cause asthma. These persons may also be allergic to peas and possibly other legumes such as soya bean oil or products, beans, or licorice. Chili beans can also be troublesome. String beans seldom cause allergy.

Nut or peanut allergies often persist throughout life in spite of diligent avoidance.

Does honey cause allergy?

The question often arises, whether honey which is gathered from plants in certain families, can cause allergies. It is generally believed that honey does not cause allergies, but it sometimes does in some patients who are acutely allergic to bee stings.

Which moulds on or in foods cause allergies?

Any food which is grown in a damp location, such as mushrooms, or aged, such as steaks, or preserved, such as smoked or pickled products, can cause symptoms. Melons, and dried or candied fruits such as apricots, raisins, and prunes can be contaminated on the outside with moulds. Certain types of cheese have moulds throughout them. Sweetened fruit beverages are sometimes unknowingly contaminated with moulds, i.e. orange juice.

Does yeast cause allergy?

Some persons cannot eat baked foods such as bread, made from a raised dough. Fermented drinks such as wine or beer can also cause difficulty. Concentrated meat extracts (Marmite) used for preparing gravy, as a beverage or a spread on toast contain high concentrations of yeast.

Can water cause allergy?

Most water is contaminated with many impurities and chemicals. Chlorine or fluorides cause symptoms in some persons. Boiling water can sometimes cause the chlorine to be expelled so it can be used. Filtering systems are also available in some countries to help purify tap water. Water-softened water also can cause symptoms in some people.

As a substitute, spring water may be suitable. Distilled water can be used but this has a bad taste. These can be used however for a few days for drinking and ALL cooking to see if this change alters the allergic symptoms.

Water can cause various allergic symptoms, but especially headaches, backaches, welts, and body swellings.

Can alcohol cause allergies?

Persons allergic to grains such as wheat, corn, barley, rye, and oats can develop allergic symptoms from drinking alcoholic beverages. Malt and hops in beer, or yeasts in beer and wine are major offenders. Champagne, in particular, can cause severe asthma in some people.

Some grass sensitive patients find they are allergic to alcohol, only during the grass pollen season, or throughout the year.

Alcohol can aggravate many forms of allergy. Intrinsic asthmatics (See page 33), persons with hay fever, and some migraine sufferers can have their symptoms made worse by alcohol. It usually does not affect young adults, unless they are mould (yeast) sensitive. Tobacco smoke in places where alcohol is served can aggravate hay fever or chest allergies.

Allergic symptoms from alcoholic drinks sometimes can be prevented by inhaling disodium cromoglycate prior to drinking. This drug, however, would not help *after* symptoms were noted. If symptoms occur, use your other allergy drugs.

Can papaya or papain cause allergy?

Papain is obtained from the fruit papaya and this is commonly used as a meat tenderizer. It is sometimes injected into animals prior to slaughter contaminating the meat so it causes symptoms when it is eaten by allergic persons. Papain is also used in medicines used to aid digestion.

Is it difficult to avoid buckwheat?

Buckwheat is difficult for allergic persons to avoid because incredibly small amounts can cause extreme reactions. Buckwheat is not wheat, but rather a weed. Some patients who are allergic to ragweed or rhubarb, have this sensitivity. The food is often eaten in the form of pancakes, Jewish kasha, or Japanese soba. Buckwheat honey or spices such as black pepper can be contaminated with it. It is used as a filler in soups or as roasted groats served with meat dishes.

The odour of buckwheat can cause allergy. Flour mills, buckwheat starched curtains, sacks of grain, Japanese pillows of buckwheat chaff, and packing material for glass items such as bulbs have been known to cause symptoms.

Similar to nut, fish, and egg sensitive persons, persons with this problem can have difficulty by indirect exposure. For example, if a wheat pancake is cooked upon a griddle which had just been used for buckwheat pancakes, a buckwheat sensitive individual could have symptoms from the wheat pancake.

WHAT OTHER PROBLEMS COULD BE RELATED TO FOOD ALLERGIES?

Can migraine headaches be triggered by allergies?

Allergy is one of many possible trigger factors related to migraine. This can be associated with eating, in particular, milk or cheese, chocolate or cola, corn, eggs, peas, beans, onions, garlic, pork, or certain spices such as cinnamon.

When cheese causes migraine, the headache is not due to an allergy to cheese but to a lack of a certain enzyme.

Other miscellaneous factors which can sometimes trigger migraine are: cigarette smoking, irritating odours, emotional upsets, fatigue, chilling, hunger, menses, and monthly hormonal changes.

Migraine headaches tend to be one-sided, located near the temple in the region between the ear and eye and forehead. Migraine is more common in women, especially if they note a significant weight increase in association with their menses. Attacks are frequently preceded by weakness, pallor, and disturbance of vision and can be associated with intestinal complaints such as nausea and vomiting. The headaches are extremely severe and prolonged, sometimes lasting days. They respond poorly to aspirin. Several members of the same family may have this difficulty. Children seldom have typical migraine headaches, but they may have a childhood form of migraine called a "migraine equivalent". This causes periodic vomiting attacks but does not cause a headache.

What is the "allergic-tension-fatigue syndrome"?

Although this is a child's syndrome, adults can have similar symptoms. It is characterized by excessive nervousness, irritability, and hyperactivity contrasted at other times by extreme fatigue, sluggishness, and listlessness. Affected persons often have vague head or muscle aches and intestinal problems. Milk, in particular, or chocolate, corn, potato, or tomato often cause it. The correct diet may cause dramatic improvement in the personality and disposition.

Patients may have other manifestations of allergies such as hay fever or asthma, but some have a personality change as their only indication of being allergic. It is not uncommon for a person's disposition to be altered after allergies develop. Fortunately a normal disposition frequently returns after the cause of the allergies has been eliminated. Use of the Multiple Food Allergy Diet (See pages 174 to 177) may quickly help eliminate a problem of this sort.

Some youngsters are so sensitive that odours of foods can cause this syndrome. Symptoms, such as irritability, have also been manifested after exposure to perfume, pollen or pets or after receiving an allergy extract treatment.

Are canker sores related to allergy?

These are painful, open, round sores usually located on the inside of the cheek or gums near the teeth. These may sometimes possibly be related to exposure to acid substances such as citric acid in the form of citrus fruits (See page 181), or by contact with acetic acid (vinegar). Apples, tomatoes, and toothpaste also have been suspected factors.

Are cold sores (herpes) caused by eating certain foods?

Cold sores are caused by activation of a herpes virus which lies dormant in certain skin areas such as the lips. When the virus is stimulated, it causes small watery painful blisters.

Fresh fruits, gum, peppermint, and chocolate are sometimes believed to activate the cold sore virus. A more common association, however, is noted whenever someone has a fever in association with a cold or infection, or when the lips are exposed to an excessive amount of sunlight or irritation.

Can ulcerative colitis be related to foods?

Chronic ulcerative colitis is rarely related to allergy. The colon part of the intestines can on occasion become inflamed because of certain foods such as milk or possibly wheat (gluten). Investigations concerning the role of allergy in this disease, as well as in some cases of other abdominal problems (gastritis and chronic pancreatitis) are presently being carried out.

Are coeliac disease and sprue allergic?

Although foods such as wheat (gluten) cause this problem, it is not due to food allergy.

CHAPTER THIRTEEN

Allergies to pets

Which pets cause allergies?

Any fur or feather covered animal can cause allergic symptoms. Common offenders are: cats, horses, dogs, birds (parakeets), hamsters, guinea pigs, mice, gerbils, rats, rabbits, chickens, goats, hogs, and cows. Direct or indirect contact with hair, saliva, dandruff (dander), urine and excreta all can cause symptoms. Cats and horses seem to cause more extreme allergic symptoms than other animals.

If a dog is frequently in a certain room, symptoms can occur when a dog allergic individual walks into the room even though the pet is not present. Hair and dandruff in the air and on the furniture can cause symptoms. Thorough cleaning is helpful, but it often takes weeks or months for symptoms to stop after removal of a pet.

Chihuahuas and poodles are said not to cause allergies because they do not shed or do not have hair. Some patients even believe that owning a chihuahua will stop their allergies. This is untrue because even a hairless dog has dandruff and saliva which can cause symptoms in certain individuals. Animal dandruff (dander) is more allergenic than hair.

Are there any pets which do not cause allergies?

If a pet has no fur or feathers, it probably will not cause allergies. Some examples are: fish, turtles, chameleons, snakes, or alligators. However, some patients are allergic to fish and have difficulty from algae or odours when they clean a fish tank, or handle fish or fish food.

Which allergic symptoms do pets cause?

Any type of symptom can be caused by a pet, for example, coughing or asthma, hay fever, eczema, or welts (nettle rash). See Chapters 2 to 5.

Are allergy skin tests for pets accurate?

A positive allergy skin test reaction usually indicates a patient is sensitive, while a negative test would mean that no allergy exists. Skin tests, however, are not always completely reliable. (See page 118). A test reaction could indicate a sensitivity to a pet sometime in the past. A positive skin test reaction often occurs in patients who have no obvious symptoms after contact with a pet. This can be noticed whenever a patient is only slightly sensitive to some allergenic substance. For example, if a small amount of grass pollen is in the air, someone might not have symptoms. A large amount of grass pollen, however, could cause that same individual to have allergies. (See page 5 re thresholds).

Skin tests with an extract made entirely from one breed of cat or dog may be inaccurate. A person can be allergic only to his own pet, to a certain breed or type of cat or dog, or to all cats and dogs. A patient may know that he is allergic to Siamese cats, while a tabby cat extract could cause a negative reaction which would give the false impression that there was no cat allergy. Such a patient would have to be tested specifically for Siamese cat to show the allergy. Unfortunately, test solutions for an individual animal or specific breeds of pets are not readily available.

Is pet allergy extract therapy effective?

There is much controversy concerning the effectiveness of extract therapy to treat pet allergies. Some allergists have found these extracts helpful. Others have not. Pet extract injection treatments can cause nose and chest symptoms of allergies in some patients. Many allergists recommend pet avoidance, rather than allergy extract injections. If patients (veterinarians or research workers) must be exposed to pets a trial period of extract therapy would be advisable.

How can rabbit contact be avoided?

In addition to avoiding rabbits, a patient should not wear rabbit trimmed or lined clothing (gloves, coats, or slippers) or rabbit fur coats which can be sold under names which would not indicate they are made from rabbits. Children should not carry rabbit's feet as good luck charms. Felt, sweaters, drapery material, upholstery and bedding can at times contain rabbit fur (See page 143). Rabbit meat probably could be eaten because it is usually well-cooked.

How can horses be avoided?

If an individual is extremely allergic to horses, contact with the animal, stables or clothing worn by persons who have been riding must be avoided. Horsehair mattresses, blankets, or clothing must not be used. Furniture can contain rubberized horsehair. It can be used to make felt or in rug pads. Cooked horse meat could cause symptoms in horse serum, dandruff or hair allergic persons unless it was well-cooked.

If a patient has only a slight reaction or sensitivity to horses, it might be possible to ride providing that horse contact occurred outside the stable and no attempt was made to brush or curry the animal. The patient should change his clothing and bathe immediately after riding.

Some patients who have a positive skin reaction to horse hair or dandruff are actually allergic to mites on the hair, and not to the horse.

How can feathers be avoided?

Birds, chickens, ducks, feather dusters or down-filled pillows, sleeping bags, comforters, or quilts are the most common forms of contact. Caged birds should not be kept in the home. The bottom of the bird cages in particular can be contaminated with mites and moulds which can cause allergy. The dust in cages is circulated as birds flap their wings.

Are most persons aware of pet allergies?

No. Persons who have symptoms immediately after cat or horse exposure, for example, know about their allergy. Many patients, however, have no obvious symptoms. Instead they wheeze or have a stuffy nose several hours after exposure.

Touching a cat or sitting in a chair where a cat rests in the afternoon could cause allergies in the middle of the night.

Whether a patient has symptoms or not is related to how allergic a patient is and how much exposure he has to a pet. For example, a non-shedding (or moulting) pet may cause no problem except when the pet is shedding or if the patient's face is licked. If a patient was very allergic, however, the slightest contact with a non-shedding animal may cause a serious reaction.

Symptoms are sometimes caused because a patient is exposed to too many allergenic substances at one time. Slight exposure to dust or exposure to dogs may not cause symptoms. Exposure to both dust and dogs on the same day, however, might cause symptoms. (See page 5).

Many patients strongly deny allergic symptoms because of their great love for their pet. When the pet is lost or dies, it is not uncommon for allergic symptoms to decrease or disappear. This may not happen for a few weeks because hair and dandruff which remains within the home may cause symptoms until the rooms are thoroughly cleaned and aired.

What happens if an allergic person keeps his pet?

The patients symptoms probably will persist. If pet contact is frequent and close, the sensitivity can become greater and symptoms could become more severe as time passes.

Many children and adults need the love and understanding which pets alone seem able to provide. Until physicians can supply pet allergy extracts which are not only entirely safe but extremely effective, there is no easy solution to the problem. The removal of a pet from a home could surely cause emotional difficulty but this effect must be weighed against the importance of keeping a family member healthy.

How can you determine the extent to which your pet causes allergic symptoms?

You can remove the pet from your home for at least one month and thoroughly clean and air your house or you can go on a holiday or visit a home which does not contain a pet for several weeks. If you notice that symptoms disappear, only to recur when you are again exposed to your personal pet, this would help to focus more directly upon the exact role which your pet plays in your symptoms.

Be careful not to assume that it must be the pet which is causing symptoms if you are better when you are away from home and worse when you return. It could be something else in your home causing difficulty. If there is doubt take your pet with you when you leave home and see if your allergies persist until you and the pet are separated.

How can you decrease pet allergies if the pet remains?

1. The best solution is to confine your pet to the outside all the time. You must consider, however, that this can be difficult for a pet if you live in a cold climate. Unless your pet runs in well-fenced in areas, the dangers of automobiles are ever present.

2. The second best answer is to confine your pet to the basement or the kitchen. The pet must *never* be allowed in the patient's bedroom, or on the furniture, or in a room in which the allergic person spends much time. If a pet is kept in the basement, a forced hot air heating system would circulate the pet's hair and dandruff throughout the home. Children should never be allowed to lie or sit directly upon a carpet if a pet is permitted in that portion of the home.

3. Allergic patients should avoid touching or contact with pets. It sometimes helps if a mask (See page 261) is used when the pet's cage is cleaned. Cleaning, grooming, and care of the pet should be carried out by non-allergic persons whenever possible.

4. Room air-purifiers or furnace units are helpful in diminishing air contamination due to pets. (See page 151). These eliminate pet dandruff and hair effectively if they are utilized in the area in which the pet is confined.

5. In some areas of the world, sprays for animals are available which can be used to help diminish shedding of hair or dandruff.

Can the development of a pet allergy be avoided?

If a person has no pet problem, infrequent contact with pets in other person's homes or outside would seldom cause an allergy to develop.

Excessive contact, however, with any animal could eventually lead to an allergy to that type of pet.

To delay or prevent the onset of a pet allergy if you own one, it would be best if the pet were kept confined to an area of the home which the patient would infrequently use. For example, if the pet were kept in a basement or in a kitchen, the dog allergy skin test may remain negative. If the pet is kept outside and contact is stringently curtailed, pet allergic symptoms will seldom develop.

Every allergist has seen patients who intentionally bring a new pet into their home. The original plan is to keep the pet confined and to keep contact sharply limited. As time passes, however, lovable pets gradually become a part of the family. The well patient notes that his symptoms reappear or new symptoms develop because of this increased contact. All in all the pet problem in the field of allergy is a most difficult one for all concerned. There is no easy simple answer except that if you have allergies, you should NOT have a pet.

If a patient has a pet allergy and the pet dies, should it be replaced?

No. If a person wants to do everything possible to prevent allergies, there should not be any pets in an allergic person's home.

When can an allergic person acquire a pet?

If a person's sole concern is to prevent allergies, no pet can be acquired until doctors have specific, effective, safe treatment for pet allergies. It is not known when or if this will be possible.

A pet sensitivity does not develop immediately after a pet is brought into a home. Pet allergies develop gradually over several months, or years. Allergic individuals may sometimes have pets and have no obvious evidence of allergies. The problem is that no one can predict what will happen. Once symptoms are caused by a pet, it is not easy to remove the pet from the home. Pets can be loved as much as children, and one simply cannot give them away or destroy them. Siblings and parents not infrequently resent the fact that an allergy in one child prevents them from bringing a pet into their home. It is difficult and unpleasant to have to choose between the health of one person and the happiness of others. Pet allergies, however, can develop in several family members. Continued repeated exposure of potentially allergic individuals to pets might eventually cause pet allergies in other family members.

Once a pet allergy develops, complete pet contact may be extremely difficult to avoid. A person who has a strong allergy to cats or dogs, for example, cannot enter a home which contains a cat or a dog. Problems arise when visiting friends and relatives or among adults whose employment necessitates visits within people's homes. Many future problems can be prevented if pet allergies are not allowed to develop.

If a pet allergy exists, can you visit relatives with pets?

The best answer is to have the relatives visit your home as much as possible, rather than the reverse. If a relative holds a cat or dog on his lap prior to visiting your home and then holds a pet allergic child, symptoms can be noticed.

During holiday seasons, in particular, relatives often visit. If a family wants to visit someone who has a pet, a few suggestions might be helpful.

1.   The person who owns the pet should place the animal outside or in a room which will seldom be used by visitors.

2.   The home should be cleaned thoroughly and aired. The walls should be wiped with a damp cloth to remove dandruff or hair attached to the walls or ceiling, and all carpeting, stuffed furniture, and draperies should be vacuumed.

3.   The patient should take prophylactic medication prior to the visit. These drugs should be continued throughout the stay providing the allergic patient does not develop progressively more severe difficulty in spite of medication.

If disodium cromoglycate (Intal), in particular, is taken *prior* to pet exposure, this often prevents symptoms from pets. This drug would be of no benefit *after* symptoms occur.

4.   An allergic person should carry his own pillow, mattress cover, blankets, and room air-purifier if he owns one.

5.   If symptoms develop in spite of all precautions during a visit to a relative, the allergic patient should leave. The family should either try to stay at a motel or return to their own home. Allergic people often become very ill when they travel.

Can visiting a zoo cause allergies?

It certainly can. Many patients who are allergic to household pets also can be allergic to other animals. For example, the lion house could cause difficulty for patients with cat allergies. The wolves might cause difficulty for patients with dog allergies.

If a person who has pet allergies stays outside the animal houses, he would have fewer symptoms than if he entered confined enclosed areas where dust and dandruff exposure would be much greater. It, also, would help to take prophylactic medication, such as disodium cromoglycate (Intal), before visiting a zoo. If symptoms arose in spite of this, the patient should leave the zoo area.

If a child with pet allergies is planning to visit a zoo with his school class, parents should acquaint the teacher with problems which might arise in their child. It might be wise to make a preliminary visit to the zoo with the youngster to be certain that no serious problems would arise. Appropriate drugs should be carried under such circumstances.

What other animal contacts cause allergic symptoms?
An individual who is allergic to animals or birds might have difficulty from the following: barns, enclosed bird sanctuaries, bull fights, circuses, cat or dog shows, farms, fair grounds, horse shows, race tracks, and stables.

CHAPTER FOURTEEN

Stinging and other insect allergy

Which insects cause allergies?

Most insect allergies are caused by stinging insects (Hymenoptera) such as bees (Apoidea), wasps, hornets, or yellow jackets (Vespoidea). Treatment for this type of allergy is excellent.

Other insects cause difficulty because they instil saliva into the skin which can cause allergic or irritating reactions. These insects include mosquitoes, flies, lice, fleas, and kissing bugs. In Africa and Asia, the sandfly (Phlebotomus) causes seasonal symptoms. The biting types of arthropods cause a small localized skin reaction but once a patient has developed an allergy, reactions are much more pronounced.

Some patients develop allergic respiratory symptoms from breathing air contaminated with insect bodies or insect excrement such as from cockroaches or locusts. The respiratory symptoms may be seasonal if the offending insect is evident only during certain months each year.

Some patients have intestinal allergic symptoms due to eating food contaminated with insects, such as cockroaches or beetles.

Some adults and many young children develop abnormally large reactions to mosquito bites. These reactions can be controlled by the use of a swallowed antihistamine and application of a skin lotion to diminish the itching. As children become older, the local reaction to mosquito bites often becomes less marked. It helps if the fingernails of young children are clean and cut very short, so that they are less apt to introduce germs or infection into the area of the bite.

When a patient develops an allergy to mosquitoes, it is possible to develop weakness, headache, fatigue, welts and an upset stomach. Such reactions are extremely rare. This type of patient possibly could be helped by treatment with mosquito allergy extract.

Deer fly, black fly, and kissing bug bites cause body swelling, coughing, wheezing, and eye and nose symptoms of allergies. Treatment of these bite reactions with allergy extracts is sometimes, but not always, effective.

Do other flies cause allergy?
All flies can cause allergic symptoms if patients are allergic to them. Some flies are found particularly near rivers or lakes. The fine scales from the wings and fly excreta, when dry, can cause acute eye irritation and nose and chest symptoms. The problem is world-wide. For example, the Nemity fly in the region of the Nile can cause acute seasonal allergic symptoms in the hot July weather.

Is it easy to identify stinging insects?
It is very difficult to identify most stinging insects. The following helps in identification of some stings. If a patient has an allergic reaction to a stinging insect, the insect should be saved and shown to your physician. If a patient is stung while walking bare-foot on the ground, the cause is frequently the large cumbersome bumble bee or the yellow jacket, because these insects nest in the ground. Honey bees are often found hovering near the ground especially if clover is evident.

There are several different types of wasps. Some wasps have no hair and a tiny "wasp" waist. Their open paper or mud combs nests are found under eaves, on porches, or in sheds. Other wasps like the hornet and yellow jacket are both hairy and often black and yellow in colour. They are all easily confused. Hornets produce football-shaped, paper-mache-like nests which usually hang from tree limbs, bushes, or under the eaves of homes.

The only insect which leaves its stinger in the victim is the honey bee.

Is an allergic individual more prone than a non-allergic individual to develop stinging insect allergies?
In some studies as many as 50 per cent of the patients who have a stinging insect allergy are found to have either a personal or family history of allergies. Normally only about 10 or possibly 20 per cent of the population has allergies. This would indicate that an allergy to stinging insects is more apt to occur in someone who has allergies, but other individuals also have this problem.

Can stinging insect reactions be fatal?
Yes. Non-fatal serious reactions are more common in children. Fatal reactions occur more often in older adults, especially in males over 30 years of age whose activities or occupations cause increased exposure. Insect stings in the ear or neck area seem to be particularly deadly.

Do all individuals have a warning reaction prior to a fatal insect sting?
Many patients do, but about 50 per cent recall no sting or advance warning in the form of any unusual previous reaction. A lack of history

of a reaction, however, does no exclude the possibility of an exquisite sensitivity to stinging insects. It is possible to develop allergy from inhaled insect dust.

If a patient has had a severe reaction to an insect sting, he is apt to have a more extreme reaction and possibly die from a subsequent sting.

Can insect stings be avoided?

The following might be helpful in diminishing the tendency to attract stinging insects:

1. Patients should wear white, tan, grey, or green clothing rather than colours or prints which are similar to flowers. Light, smooth clothing is preferable to dark rough fabrics. Insects should not confuse people with flowers. Persons who have stinging insect allergies should neither look nor smell like a flower.

2. A liquid insect repellent can be helpful. This can be applied to clothing, hair, or exposed body parts. It should be used on picnics or occasions when the patient will be in an area where there could be stinging insects. It is helpful if a rapid acting insecticide is kept in a family automobile and at a patient's bedside.

3. Allergic individuals should avoid cutting lawns, picking flowers, playing in bushes, trimming hedges, disposing of garbage, or walking through clover, garden areas, orchards of ripe fruit, greenhouses, boat docks, or abandoned old buildings.

Attics or eaves in homes can be a nesting area for stinging insects, and persons can be stung during the cold or winter months. Curious youngsters should be warned never to tamper with stinging insect nests or to touch struggling, drowning insects on the surface of water such as a swimming pool.

4. Shoes which adequately cover the feet should be worn. For example, patients should not walk barefoot or wear sandals when walking on grass or near clover.

5. Persons with stinging insect allergies should avoid using nicely scented substances which might attract insects. This would include hair spray or dressing, deodorant, body powder, scented soap, perfume, lotion, or carrying scented facial tissue.

6. Jewellery and perspiration are possible factors which can attract insects.

7. Loose fitting clothing should not be worn because stinging insects can become trapped in folds of cloth, such as long dresses or wide-legged trousers.

8. Any stinging insect nests near the patient's home should be removed by exterminators. Under no circumstance should a patient allergic to stinging insects attempt to solve this problem on his own.

9. Persons with this allergy should not have bee hives or raise bees.

What is a normal reaction to a stinging insect?

The site of the sting normally causes pain, itching, and becomes swollen. Some patients repeatedly have extremely large reactions to stinging insects, but do not develop any problem which affects areas of the body distant from the sting. If a sting, for example, occurs on the elbow it may cause the arm to swell from the shoulder to the wrist but it should not cause swelling or *any* reaction on *any* other portion of the body such as the face, leg, back, or other arm.

What is the usual treatment for a normal reaction to a stinging insect?

If a venom sac is left in the skin, it should be removed. Care should be taken to flick it out with a fingernail in such a way that more venom is not squeezed into the skin. A paste of meat tenderizer and water or ice can be applied to help diminish the localized pain and swelling. Aspirin (or an aspirin-substitute) and an antihistamine may help to decrease pain. itching, and swelling.

Do extremely large local reactions to stinging insects need treatment with allergy injection treatments?

There is no uniform agreement among allergists concerning this. Many do not treat extreme local reactions, while others believe that certain selected patients should be treated. There is no way to predict which severe local reactions will precede a future alarming allergic reaction.

What is a definite abnormal reaction to a stinging insect?

Any immediate or delayed reaction to a stinging insect which affects a portion of the body *distant from the sting site* should be considered abnormal. Immediate non-fatal abnormal reactions usually last less than 3 days. This type of reaction could be manifested by welts (nettle rash) or swelling in some area of the body other than the site of the sting; or by eye, nose, or chest symptoms of allergies.

Some patients also have intestinal upsets, shock, weakness, nausea, dizziness, a hoarse voice, throat swelling, confusion, feelings of anxiety and even unconsciousness with loss or urine and bowel contents. Eczema has been noted subsequent to some reactions.

Patients who die from allergic insect sting reactions generally have breathing problems because of swelling of the upper windpipe or larynx. Sometimes, however, the patient has a shock-like reaction (faint and become pale) or haemorrhage. Heart failure and infarcts have been noted especially in older persons suggesting that circulatory problems can predispose individuals to a possible fatal reaction to an insect sting.

What should an untreated patient do for an abnormal reaction to an insect sting?

If a venom sac is evident, it should be removed using a flicking motion, not squeezed. Apply a tourniquet between the sting and the rest of the body if the sting occurred on the arms or the legs. Ice should be placed on the region of the sting. If the patient has an antihistamine and a drug to treat asthma, *both* should be given immediately. Because these would not help for 10 or 15 minutes, most patients also carry adrenaline for injection or an adrenaline-like inhaler or spray to use for an emergency allergic reaction. If either is used, contact your physician immediately or go to the nearest hospital.

Stinging insect allergy patients should *always* carry an antihistamine and asthma drugs for emergency use until they have been well-immunized for this problem.

Stinging insect emergency kits can be prepared. These should contain a tourniquet, a syringe, some adrenaline, an antihistamine, and an ephedrine tablet. Cortisone is usually not helpful because it would require serveral hours to give relief. In order to use a syringe correctly a patient would have to check with his physician concerning the correct dosage of adrenaline and how to inject it.

Speed is essential in treating an abnormal reaction. Fatalities are definitely less if a patient receives treatment as soon as possible. Because fatalities can occur within a few minutes, it is essential that each patient be prepared completely to treat any stinging insect emergency.

Patients should always carry a card in their wallet or wear a name tag stating that they have a stinging insect allergy. Such identification could conceivably save a patient's life because medical personnel would make a correct diagnosis more quickly if a patient were unconscious at the time of arrival at a hospital.

Anyone who has an abnormal reaction to a stinging insect, must be seen by a physician (or allergist) so that skin testing and allergy extract treatment can be started. This form of treatment is very effective and is mandatory for any mild or severe, generalized stinging insect reaction.

Should adrenaline-like drugs be used by injection or aerosol?

Either an injection or aerosol spray of adrenaline can be used to treat an allergic stinging insect emergency. Adrenaline for injection should be observed often and replaced if it changes from colourless to brown because this indicates that it has oxidized. If adrenaline is allowed to remain in a hot area, it can turn brown very quickly.

The exact dosage of adrenaline (1:1000) for injection should be determined by your physician. In general, 0.2 ml. is the dosage administered to a (20 kg.) four-year-old. An adult could receive approximately 0.3 or 0.4 ml. The correct dose can be repeated twice, if 15 minutes elapses between each dose.

Stinging insect allergy patients should be careful to keep a stinging insect emergency kit at home, at work or school, and in the family car.

Because an adrenaline-like aerosol will stimulate the heart, as will an injection of adrenaline, these two drugs should *not* be taken by a patient at exactly the same time. Patients who are having an allergic emergency should use one or the other, as advised by their physician.

An adrenaline-like aerosol spray is similar to an injection of adrenaline but it is much easier to carry. It sometimes can help a patient breathe more easily within seconds provided the spray is properly used. (See page 107).

What is a toxic reaction to an insect sting?

This type of reaction often occurs when an individual is stung by several, usually 10 or more, insects. Swelling, with or without welts (nettle rash), headache, fever, drowsiness, weakness, muscle spasm, convulsions, and dizziness can occur. Some of these symptoms might not occur for several hours.

At times it is difficult to tell the difference between a toxic and an allergic reaction. The toxic reaction is due to the injection of too much toxin or venom, whereas an allergic reaction is due to an abnormal sensitivity to the venom. The exact diagnosis should be made by your physician.

Can a patient have a delayed reaction to a stinging insect?

A delayed allergic reaction rarely occurs but sometimes patients do not have symptoms for several hours or up to 10 days after an insect sting. Most serious reactions occur in less than 6 hours. The delayed type of reaction can cause a fever, upset stomach, weakness, joint pain, hives, lymph node swelling in the armpits, groin or neck, nervous system problems, or bleeding into the skin or bowels.

Very rarely patients have a typical immediate allergic reaction to an insect sting and in addition, several days later, develop delayed symptoms. If a patient has no symptoms within 10 to 14 days after an insect sting, it is most doubtful that problems will be noted.

Some, but not all, allergists believe that patients who have delayed reactions should be treated with stinging insect extract injections.

How should a patient be treated if he is stung *after* he has received stinging insect extract therapy?

Patients who have been *adequately* treated with stinging insect extract seldom need to receive any particular treatment when they are stung. If symptoms are noted, however, or if there is concern, they should take an antihistamine, a drug to treat asthma, some form of adrenaline, and see a physician as soon as possible.

When patients are receiving their extract at an interval of 4 weeks or more, it usually indicates that they are receiving the maximum amount of extract. Each top dosage of stinging extract, is roughly equal to at least 2 or 3 stings from a stinging insect.

If a patient previously received treatment for stinging insects but stopped his allergy extract injections, the sensitivity can recur. If this happens, the patient should immediately re-start his allergy extract therapy for stinging insects. Until this is done, he should carry prophylactic drugs at all times. (See page 202).

If a well-treated patient is stung by many stinging insects at one time, allergy drugs in the form of an antihistamine and an asthma drug should be taken immediately. Hope for the best, expect the worst, and immediately go to a hospital.

How much time can elapse between a sting and a fatal reaction?

Fatalities generally occur *in less than* 15 minutes, although sometimes death occurs within the first hour. It is for this reason that a patient must be prepared to cope with the emergency situation *on his own.* There may not be adequate time to secure the help of a physician, especially if the patient were unconscious in less than 5 minutes. Parents of young children must watch their child carefully and be certain that babysitters or relatives who care for the child know *exactly* how to handle an insect sting reaction.

In general, the shorter the interval of time between the sting and the onset of the symptoms, the more severe the reaction will be. If no reaction is evident other than at the site of the sting after a period of 30 to 60 minutes, it is unlikely (but not impossible) that a reaction will occur.

Can a well treated stinging insect allergic patient expire from a sting?

This is possible but fortunately treatment failures are rare. In most patients, stinging insect immunization is very effective.

Does pollen on a stinging insect cause allergic reactions?

It is not the pollen on the stinger or the insect's body which causes this allergy. It is a reaction to the venom which is injected into the patient's body. However, there are patients who are so extremely sensitive that eating honey or going near to a beehive can cause reactions.

Does skin testing help diagnose stinging insect allergy?

The skin test sensitivity may or may not parallel the actual allergy.

Sometimes a patient has a completely negative skin test reaction although the history indicates a strong stinging insect allergy. Patients who have this type of response are sometimes treated regardless of the skin test results. Each patient's care must be individualized.

When should skin tests for stinging insects be carried out?

It is possible to have a negative reaction to a stinging insect test during the first week or two after a sting. For this reason, it is more reliable to be skin tested 2 weeks after a sting has occurred.

Because there is a similarity among the different stinging insects, many doctors skin test and treat with a combination of several stinging insects, rather than for individual ones. For example, it is possible to have a severe allergic reaction to a wasp sting. A subsequent sting from a honey bee in some individuals may or may not cause the same allergic reaction. Treatment with several types of stinging insects can avoid this problem. The physician in charge should make the final decision.

How effective is stinging insect injection therapy?

According to some studies as many as 94 per cent of patients are helped. An exceptional patient, however, might have more severe reactions in spite of extract therapy. At the present time it is recommended that stinging insect allergic patients receive treatments indefinitely. The interval between injection treatments, however, can gradually be increased in some patients after 2 or 3 years of therapy. Patients who stop their treatments sometimes die from subsequent stings!

CHAPTER FIFTEEN

Allergies to drugs

Which common drugs cause allergies?
Any medicine can cause an allergy or hypersensitivity reaction. Major offenders are:
Aspirin
Antibiotics – such as penicillin, sulfonamides or sulfa drugs, and tetracyclines
Skin Drugs
Local Anesthetics
Iodides or Bromides
Anticonvulsive Drugs
Hormones – such as insulin or ACTH
Tranquillizers – such as phenothiazines
Laxatives – such as phenolphthalein
Sedatives containing barbiturates – such as phenobarbital
Narcotic Drugs – such as codeine or morphine
Alcohol
Vaccines
Contraceptives
Vitamins
Nose Drops
Lozenges

What types of reactions occur from drug allergies?
Typical reactions include skin rashes, welts, body swelling, hay fever, or asthma. Less frequent reactions are drug fever, lymph node swelling, changes in the liver, lungs, or kidney, or alterations in the blood.

What are photosensitivity reactions?
These reactions are due to an interaction of a drug and sunlight. A rash appears on the skin areas exposed to sunlight. The rash looks like a severe sunburn, but may be caused by minimal exposure to light. Sun-

light must be avoided or sunscreen lotions must be used for several weeks for this type of problem.

Allergy is responsible for specific types of photosensitivity reactions. These reactions can be caused by some antibiotics, skin medications (coal tars), tranquillizers, diuretics, or oral diabetic drugs. Drugs causing a photosensitivity reaction must be avoided. Medicated shampoos may be a common cause of a sun rash called a solar dermatitis.

How can you determine if a drug is causing an undesirable effect?

Many sick patients take several drugs at the same time. Drugs may cause major problems or mild undesirable effects such as nausea, headache, irritability or fatigue. Your physician may be able to tell you which drug is most apt to cause common problems without any particular investigation. For example, certain antibiotics often cause an itchy genital or rectal area (See page 97). If the problem is not easily solved, your doctor may be able to advise you how to check each individual drug to determine if any caused an undesirable effect.

Is there a way to skin-test for drug allergies?

Skin tests can be performed to help detect some drug allergies. These tests are often helpful in diagnosing penicillin allergy and sometimes of value in diagnosing insulin or ACTH allergy. Skin tests for drugs can, however, be misleading.

Even though there are different ways to test a patient's skin or blood, for example, for penicillin allergy, it is not always possible to make a completely accurate diagnosis. Someone may be sensitive to penicillin but have no reaction to the drug skin test. Another patient may have a strong positive penicillin reaction but have no problem from this drug. Usually, however, persons with positive tests are allergic to the drug. Many persons believe themselves to be allergic to penicillin when they are not.

Although intensive research is being carried out in the field of drug allergy detection at the present time there have been very few major breakthroughs. We cannot, for example, accurately detect an allergy to aspirin, phenobarbital, most antibiotics, or iodides used to X-ray kidneys, gall bladder, or blood vessels. It is anticipated that more accurate detection of drug allergies will be possible eventually.

Are allergic individuals more prone to drug allergies than other persons?

Anyone can develop a drug allergy. There is no convincing evidence that these reactions occur more often in allergic persons. Allergic persons, however, are more apt to have *serious* allergic reactions to drugs. This is especially true in relation to penicillin. Children have fewer allergies to drugs such as penicillin or aspirin, than do adults.

Many individuals falsely believe they are allergic to a certain drug because a possible reaction occurred during or subsequent to the use of a drug. Until we have more accurate testing methods, patients must be wary of using *any* drug to which they are *believed* to be allergic. Drug reactions are most common in persons who have chronic diseases because they have more drug exposure. Persons who have one drug hypersensitivity are more prone to develop new drug allergies.

Some allergists prophylactically recommend that all allergic persons avoid the use of penicillin and aspirin in an effort to prevent the development of sensitivity to these common drugs.

How soon after taking a drug can an allergic reaction occur?

Reactions often occur immediately or while a drug is being taken, but sometimes difficulty might not be noted until after the drug has been stopped. It is possible, for example, to take a drug such as penicillin for 6 days but not begin to react until the 9th day, even though the drug had not been used for 3 days.

If an individual is using several drugs at the time of a typical drug reaction, all of these might have to be discontinued temporarily. A physician's aid would help in detecting which drug most probably caused the allergic reaction.

Once a drug reaction begins, how long does it last?

Drug reactions can last for a few hours, days, or even months. If a certain drug causes a rash, the rash often starts to fade within a few hours after the drug is stopped. Under some circumstances, however, the rash could last for several weeks. Penicillin reactions, at times, may recur or last for many months because of penicillin contact in disguised forms. Farmers sometimes treat udder infections (mastitis) in cows with penicillin causing contamination of milk and dairy products.

Which recommendations might help drug allergic patients?

1.   You need to know the exact name of the drug which causes the reaction, and you must be certain to remind both the physician and chemist that you have this allergy so that it is not prescribed in an unrecognized form.

2.   You should always carry a card in your wallet or wear some identification stating which particular drug causes allergy.

Why should a patient carry identification concerning drug allergies?

Many parents do not feel very young children need to wear a name tag about a drug allergy because adult supervision is always present. A problem can arise, however, when children are cared for by babysitters, neighbours, or friends and need emergency treatment. It would be essential that the emergency room physician know about the youngsters' exact allergies. Children should have this information on a wrist or necklace type name tag.

Adults may believe drug allergy identification to be unnecessary because they know the drugs to which they are allergic. Accidents, however, can happen causing unconsciousness or confusion.

Which drug reactions are not due to allergies?

If a reaction occurs after using a drug, it does not mean that it is caused by an allergy. Certain drugs may cause repeated diarrhoea because of bowel irritation. This may be only an undesirable side effect. If a drug helps and the undesirable side effect is not severe, it may be possible to continue using the drug. Problems of this sort, however, should be discussed with your physician.

Some patients are "intolerant" of certain drugs. This means that they cannot tolerate the usual dosage of a drug. For example, massive doses of aspirin can cause an upset stomach, ringing in the ears, and dizziness. If, however, a patient takes a recommended dosage of aspirin and develops nausea, dizziness, and ear ringing, this is called intolerance.

A true allergy to a drug causes symptoms which in no way are related to the usual response to an excessive amount of that particular drug. For example, if one aspirin tablet causes a nettle rash, this could be an allergy. If one aspirin, however, causes ringing in the ears, this is an intolerance.

Some drugs can cause problems which are not due to a side effect, or intolerance, or an allergy. For example, they may cause a marked decrease in the number of white blood cells making a patient prone to develop infection. Liver or kidney damage can be noted after the use or misuse of certain drugs. Sometimes enzymes, essential for normal body function, may be lacking after the use of certain drugs. These reactions are sometimes related to an idiosyncrasy to a medication.

What is aspirin?

Aspirin is acetylsalicylic acid. It is the acetyl part of the drug which causes medical problems, although some patients also have difficulty from salicylates.

How should a headache be treated if aspirin cannot be used?

Aspirin substitutes are available. These medicines contain paracetamol rather than acetyl salicylic acid (aspirin). Sodium salicylate may not cause symptoms in some patients who cannot use aspirin.

Are aspirin reactions due to allergy?

Reactions to aspirin are called hypersensitivity, rather than an allergy because the exact mechanisms by which these occur cannot be adequately explained. Allergy skin tests for aspirin are not of value.

Aspirin sensitive individuals should never use the smallest amount of aspirin. If such persons merely place an aspirin tablet on the tongue, it might cause immediate death.

Which symptoms are associated with aspirin hypersensitivity?

Swellings within the nose called polyps are frequently evidenced, as well as asthma, sinus infections, welts (nettle rash), body swellings, and bleeding problems.

What are nasal polyps?

Polyps are moist, smooth, bluish-white swellings within the nose which look like a grape which has been skinned. Chronic irritation or infection within the nose, such as the sinuses, can cause these swellings to become red, rough, or wrinkled. Because other growths can cause blockage in the nose, patients who have polyps should *always* be seen by an ear, nose, and throat physician.

These growths are noted mainly in adults who may or may not have had nose allergies. Children rarely have polyps unless they have had a chronic infection within the nose or cystic fibrosis. Polyps seldom occur in young children.

Polyps rarely disappear spontaneously and often have to be removed repeatedly by surgery. Some doctors are reluctant to do this during a pollen season because, as with any surgery of the nose or throat, asthma may be precipitated. If polyps are in part related to allergy, proper allergic management and removal of offending substance is essential to help prevent their recurrence.

Some patients have a combination of nose polyps, infection, asthma and aspirin sensitivity. Although such patients can have allergic-type blood cells (eosinophils) in their blood or nose and lung mucus, the common causes of typical allergy do not seem to be a factor related to this particular combination of symptoms.

Is anything typical of aspirin-induced asthma?

Patients who have this problem are often middle-aged and have had nose symptoms, associated with nasal polyps, for several or many years. Asthma may not occur until the individual is 40 or 50 years old and the initial attack is often associated with a respiratory infection. Asthma may occur within 2 hours after taking aspirin. The asthma attacks are severe and extremely difficult to control. (See page 83 re operations).

Which miscellaneous items can possibly cause hypersensitivity reactions in persons allergic to salicylates?
   The following may or do contain salicylates and could possibly cause problems for some aspirin sensitive patients:

FLAVOURING

Antiseptics	Beverages	Cosmetics	Candles
Gum	Mouthwash	Toothpaste	Perfumes
Lozenges	Oil of Wintergreen		

Foods that contain salicylates in flavouring: ice cream, bakery goods (except bread), candy, chewing gum, soft drinks, gelatin, and jams.

FOODS

Almonds	Currants	Peaches	Strawberries
Apples	Gooseberries	Plums	Birch beer
Apricots	Grapes	Prunes	Teaberry Tea
Blackberries	Nectarines	Raisins	Wines
Cherries	Oranges	Raspberries	Wine Vinegar

PLANTS

Aspens	Willows	Calvanthus	Milkwort
Birches	Acacia	Camellia	Tulips
Poplars	Spiraea	Hyacinth	Violets
	Teaberry	Marigold	

MISCELLANEOUS

Acetyl salicylic acid	Acid (in lubricating oils)	Salicylsalicylic acid
Aluminum acetyl salicylate	Methyl salicylate	Santyl (santyl salicylate)
Ammonium salicylate	Para amino salicylic acid	Soap (green, winter-green fragrance)
Arthropan	Phenyl salicylate	Stroncylate
Calcium acetyl salicylate	Procaine salicylate	Strontium salicylate
Choline salicylate	Sal ethyl carbonate	Sulfosalicylic acid (chemical)
Ethyl salicylate	Salicylamide	Suntan lotions
Lithium salicylate	Salicylanilide (anti-mildew)	
Methylene disalicylic		

Can patients not realize they are aspirin sensitive?
Yes. Many persons are totally unaware of their aspirin sensitivity. For example, many patients wheeze with most infections. At the first sign of infection, aspirin is often taken for fever or pain. The aspirin can cause wheezing which the patient incorrectly attributes to infection.
If aspirin is taken and no wheeze is noted within 2 or 3 hours, an aspirin sensitivity is unlikely. If you think you are sensitive to aspirin, do not try to take one without your physician's supervision.
Any cold, headache, or pain drug can contain aspirin. Persons sensitive to aspirin must read the labels of any drugs which they purchase carefully to be certain they contain no acetyl-salicylic acid.

Can a diabetic become allergic to insulin?
This can happen. The problem may be easily solved by changing brands of insulin, or by using a form of insulin which is made from pigs (porcine) rather than from cows (bovine). Insulin preparations can be altered by heating so they retain their effectiveness but do not cause an allergic reaction. This problem requires the assistance of a physician. Some patients may react to all types of insulin. If insulin treatment is necessary, careful desensitization with gradually stronger amounts of insulin can be attempted cautiously by specialist physicians.

Do iodide preparations cause allergy?
Iodides cause two major types of reactions. The first type is not an allergy but a side effect often noted after taking an iodide to thin mucus (an expectorant). Common side effects are an acne-like rash (located on any part of the body), enlargement of the saliva glands, swollen tearing red eyes, a watery nose, a sore throat, a husky voice, or possibly a tender underactive thyroid gland. These reactions often disappear completely when the iodide medicine is discontinued.
The second type is a hypersensitivity reaction which could cause a drug fever, welts, skin rashes, or swollen joints.
One other problem is due to the dark brown colour of iodides. Staining of the teeth can occur. Teeth should be brushed vigorously after taking liquid medicine which contains iodides.
Iodides are sometimes used to X-ray the kidneys (intravenous pyelograms), heart (angiocardiogram), or inside of the lungs (bronchograms). Unfortunately, there is no safe reliable way to test for an iodide sensitivity before it is used. Some physicians recommend that persons who have developed a rash or hives after iodides avoid having X-rays taken with an iodide-like drug. Reactions to iodinated material can occur in patients who have no allergies and may *not* occur in some persons who have had undesirable side effects from iodides.
The exact mechanism of iodide reactions, similar to aspirin reactions

are not well understood. There is evidence that such a sensitivity is not typically allergic.

Can an individual be allergic to a fluoride?
There have been some reported sensitivities to this chemical when it has been added to tooth paste, vitamin preparations, or water.

Can drugs which contain mercury cause allergies?
This is possible. The slightest exposure to items which contain mercury can cause severe reactions in persons who are sensitive to it. Ointments and certain antiseptics to reduce infections can contain mercury. Mercury compounds are frequently used in eye or ear ointments or drops, in some types of tooth filling and in certain diuretics. Reactions to mercurials often cause a skin rash and may cause headache, nausea, joint pains, and other problems.

Do quinine products cause allergies?
The reactions to quinine products in sensitive individuals can appear in many forms and are not necessarily allergic. For example, some patients have dizziness, ringing in their ears, hearing or visual problems, intestinal upsets, bleeding, welts or body swelling, or nervousness.

Quinine is sometimes used in treating heart disorders or malaria. It is used in mixed drinks which contain quinine or tonic water. If a patient likes gin and tonic, he must dilute the gin with something other than tonic water.

Do barbiturates or sedatives cause allergies?
Five per cent of patients who use barbiturates develop sensitivity reactions mainly in the form of a skin rash, nettle rash or welts, or fever. Innumerable drugs used to treat asthma may contain small amounts of barbiturates. Great care must be taken if a barbiturate allergy exists. One barbiturate reaction is called a *fixed drug reaction*. This means that each time the drug is taken, a rash appears in the *same* area of the skin.

What is a paraben allergy?
Paraben substances cause skin rashes and are frequently found in cosmetics such as lotions, creams, or ointments. Patients who have this sensitivity can also react to parabens found in some foods, in teeth cleaning preparations, and in suppositories. Dermatologists can diagnose this problem by using patch tests.

Do local anaesthetics cause allergy?
Anaesthetics used in dentistry cause relatively few reactions but this

type of sensitivity can occur in some patients. The reaction can occur immediately or several hours after a local anaesthetic has been injected for dental repair. Skin testing for these drugs has not been found to be helpful.

There are two major groups of local anaesthetics. If an individual is allergic to a member of one group, he may have difficulty from similar drugs in that group. Unrelated drugs in a second group may cause no problems. One group includes drugs such as benzocaine, monocaine, clorprocaine, and tetracaine. The other group includes lidocaine (xylocaine), and phenacaine.

Which suggestions might help a person sensitive to local anaesthetics?
1.   The patient can have the dentist use a local anaesthetic drug in a chemical group different from the one causing the reaction.
2.   The patient should have dental care without the use of any anaesthetic, if possible.
3.   He might try nitrous oxide but all patients cannot tolerate this gas.
4.   Hypnosis can be tried to relieve pain from dental repair.

Local anaesthetics are used not only for dental procedures but are also used for minor surgery requiring anaesthesia of a small area of skin.

It is possible for patients allergic to certain "caine" products, such as benzocaine, to be allergic to sulfonamide-type drugs.

What is an antibiotic?
An antibiotic is a drug used to treat infection. There are several different types of antibiotics, i.e. penicillin, tetracyclines, and erythromycins. Other drugs used to treat infections are called chemotherapeutic agents, such as sulfonamides. Antibiotics kill or hinder the growth of bacteria, or germs which cause infection. Select types of bacteria are eliminated by different antibiotics. Some infections are not stopped until the correct antibiotic is given. It may be necessary to grow or culture the exact germ which is causing an infection in order to determine exactly which antibiotic is best. The common cold or other viral infections are not helped by antibiotics, because we have no drugs to treat these infections. Excellent antiviral agents, however, are available to treat herpes viral infections (like cold sores).

How significant is diarrhoea caused by an antibiotic?
Mild diarrhoea is not important, providing the infection is eliminated by the antibiotic. If the diarrhoea is a severe significant problem, a physician must be contacted.

Diarrhoea indicates that the bowel has been irritated. If it is a minor problem, the diarrhoea may be eliminated by lowering the dose of the antibiotic as suggested by your physician.

Which antibiotics cause allergies?
   Any antibiotics can cause an allergy. Penicillin and sulfonamide possibly cause more allergic reactions than other antibiotics. Penicillin is broken down in the body into many different chemicals and an individual can be allergic to one or more of these altered penicillin forms.
The following antibiotics also frequently cause allergic reactions:
   1.   Streptomycin
   2.   Neomycin – approximately 5 to 10 per cent of individuals are allergic to this drug. This drug is used mainly in skin ointments, creams, and eye drops. (See page 63).
   3.   Tetracycline – can cause skin rashes. Certain types tend to cause a photosensitivity reaction.
   Tetracyclines can cause other problems. In some children, who take this type of drug before the age of 7 or 8 years, it can permanently cause the adult teeth to be discoloured either a bluish grey or brownish tan colour. This can be noticed as soon as the adult teeth appear.
   4.   Chloromycetin is infrequently used because it can cause serious blood changes in some patients. It also can cause a fever or skin rash.
   5.   Cephalothins are drugs which are used sometimes by persons who are allergic to penicillin. Unfortunately occasional penicillin allergic patients are sometimes also allergic to the cephalothins. A cephalothin sensitivity can damage blood cells.
   One of the safest antibiotic drugs available is erythromycin. Few allergic reactions have been reported to it, although on occasion, individuals do develop skin rashes, diarrhoea, or even jaundice.
   Unfortunately, some individuals are allergic to several antibiotics, and treatment of infection becomes a major problem. When new drugs are used in such individuals the dosage should be relatively small initially. Antibiotics should not be used unless your physician advises that they are essential. The fewer antibiotics a patient uses, the less chance there will be for reactions and the development of antibiotic allergies.

What is a monilial (yeast or Candida) infection?
   This type of infection is frequently seen after the use of many types of antibiotics. Antibiotics tend to destroy the normal bacteria or germs which are found in the intestines. When these normal bacteria are eliminated, there tends to be an overgrowth of the remaining yeast-like organisms called monilia or Candida.
   For example, sometimes individuals who use antibiotics develop

itching around the rectum, or in the region of the vagina, caused by monilia. Special drugs are needed to eliminate this type of yeast.

What can you do if you need the drug to which you are allergic?
This type of problem frequently arises when a patient is allergic to penicillin. Penicillin may be the best or even only drug to treat a certain infection.
The physician and patient may be faced with a dilemma. If penicillin is not given, a disease might be fatal. If the antibiotic is given, the patient could become very ill from the penicillin which could cause a serious allergic reaction. The physician must weigh the potential danger of the disease against the possible adverse effects from treatment. A specialist is often needed to help in determining exactly when and how penicillin treatments can be given under such circumstances. Frequent small doses, given with great care and caution, are sometimes possible even though someone is allergic to penicillin.
There is now such a wide range of antibiotics from which to choose that one can often be recommended which has never been received previously. If a patient is dangerously allergic to many antibiotics, it is a good rule to admit the patient to the hospital. With constant skilled care, no antibiotic may be necessary.

Do some antibiotic allergies tend to occur in certain families?
Yes. It is not unusual, for example, for several members of one family to be sensitive to a certain drug such as penicillin. If a problem of this sort is noted, other family members should avoid the use of this drug so that they do not become allergic to it.

Is it possible to be allergic to vaccines used to immunize children or adults?
This is certainly possible. See page 221 for more information.

Do blood transfusions cause special problems in allergic persons?
When an individual receives a blood transfusion, the blood which the patient is to receive, is carefully compared with his own to be certain that there is no major incompatibility. Persons who have allergies, however, to drugs or foods, can definitely have difficulty after receiving blood from individuals who recently have been in contact with these particular items. For example, an individual who is very sensitive to fish could have a marked allergic reaction if he were transfused with the blood of a person who had recently eaten fish. Similarly, if an individual received blood containing penicillin when he was allergic to penicillin, a reaction could occur.
It is even possible to cause allergic symptoms in non-allergic indivi-

duals. For example, suppose someone has never had difficulty from grass pollen. If this person receives blood from someone whose hay fever is due to grass pollen, during the time when grass pollen is in the air, the non-allergic person could develop hay fever. For the above reason, in some countries, persons who have allergies are ineligible for blood donations.

CHAPTER SIXTEEN

Immunizations and allergy

Which immunizations cause *no* difficulty in allergic individuals?

Persons with allergies have no *particular* or *special* problems when they receive immunization treatments against diphtheria, tetanus (lockjaw), pertussis (whooping cough), rubella (German measles), polio, or cholera. On rare occasions, however, any individual can develop a reaction to any vaccine.

If a particular adult or child has an untoward reaction to any of the above vaccines, it is sometimes possible to immunize him either by using a different brand name of vaccine or by having the vaccine given in small amounts on several occasions, rather than giving the total recommended dosage at one time.

Which forms of immunization can cause difficulty in allergic persons?

Different types of immunization vaccines are grown on various types of tissues, such as chick, rabbit or dog. Anyone who develops obvious allergic symptoms from contact with eggs, chickens, or feathers should avoid any vaccine grown on chick or avian (bird or duck) tissue culture. Persons who have obvious allergic symptoms from exposure to dogs or rabbits should not receive vaccines grown on dog or rabbit tissue culture. Individuals who know they have a neomycin allergy (See page 215) should avoid any vaccine which contains this type of antibiotic.

It is important, however, to remember that a positive allergy skin test reaction to dogs, eggs, chickens, rabbits and feathers is of *no* significance in relation to immunization. It is only of importance if someone has obvious symptoms when he is exposed to the item which is used to produce the vaccine.

To further confuse the issue, there are studies which indicate that although some patients are very sensitive to contact with eggs or dogs, they can be safely immunized with vaccines prepared on egg or dog media. Immunization, however, of persons with this type of sensitivity should not be routinely recommended and the advice of a specialist should be secured if this question arises in relation to any particular patient.

Are there special precautions related to different vaccines?
The vaccines available in different countries throughout the world will not be alike. In some countries, the same vaccine may be grown upon different types of tissue depending upon which drug company makes it. If a patient, for example, cannot tolerate eggs, he should ask his physician if he can secure vaccine grown upon a type of tissue to which he is not sensitive. Some vaccines may be filtered through silk, contain antibiotics such as penicillin or neomycin, or preservatives such as phenol or mercurials. Any of these could cause symptoms in sensitive persons.

A.   RUBEOLA OR MEASLES VACCINE

In Great Britain, this vaccine is obtained from material grown on chicken tissues. Measles vaccine, like some influenza vaccine, has been known to cause an allergic asthmatic child to have more asthma for the next month or so. Although measles is undesirable because it can affect the lungs, it would seem better to allow the child to have an attack of measles even if the asthmatic child were on cortisone treatment. Surprisingly most asthmatic children are no more upset by measles than the non-asthmatic. In any outbreak of measles there will be a few children who become very ill with various complaints, but most children have little difficulty.

B.   RUBELLA OR GERMAN MEASLES

In Great Britain, this vaccine is available from rabbit tissue cultures. It may contain neomycin.

C.   MUMPS VACCINE

In Great Britain this is grown on chicken tissue. It may also contain neomycin.

D.   SMALLPOX VACCINE

This vaccine should not be received by persons who have eczema, burns, impetigo, or skin problems unless so advised by their physician.
Persons who are receiving cortisone or similar drugs should not be vaccinated.
Some countries no longer require routine smallpox immunizations.

E. INFLUENZA VACCINE

This is most frequently grown on egg or chicken tissue material. Some health services in some countries recommend that persons who have asthma or chronic lung disease receive this vaccine each year. The vaccine is usually given several months before influenza is usually apparent in a community. You can check with your public health service to determine the recommendations in the area in which you live. There is evidence that an injection of (killed) influenza vaccine makes many allergic asthmatic children have increased symptoms for one to three months. It is wise, therefore, not to attempt to protect a child with asthma against influenza unless so advised by your physician.

F. TYPHUS VACCINE

This is most frequently grown on an egg culture.

G. POLIOMYELITIS VACCINE

Injectable polio vaccine sometimes contains preservatives or antibiotics such as penicillin which can cause allergic reactions in certain individuals. Oral polio vaccine eliminates this problem.

H. PLAGUE VACCINE

This vaccine sometimes can cause welts or nettle rash on the arms.

I. YELLOW FEVER VACCINE

This vaccine is grown on chicken egg material and could possibly cause a reaction in patients who could not eat eggs.

J. RABIES VACCINE

This vaccine is grown on rabbit or duck tissue.

How do tetanus-toxoid and tetanus-antitoxin differ?

A toxin is a poison produced by bacteria such as the ones causing tetanus or lockjaw. A toxoid is routinely injected into adults and children so protection is made by their bodies against lockjaw or tetanus. This is tetanus immunization. If it is received at recommended intervals, patients exposed to tetanus usually will have or can readily make adequate protection to prevent lockjaw.

In contrast, tetanus antitoxin is a special serum which is obtained from the blood of animals who have received tetanus-toxoid and developed protection against lockjaw. If horse tetanus antitoxin is injected into an injured patient, it provides that person with *immediate* protection against tetanus. Although tetanus antitoxin is usually given in the form of horse serum, it is also available from cow serum or human serum.

How often should a person receive tetanus-toxoid (lockjaw) immunization?

The recommendations of physicians vary in different countries, and in the same country at different times. In general, tetanus toxoid is recommended approximately 3 times during the first year of life, and at varying intervals from then on.

The protection from a vaccine lasts a considerable number of years in many people. Adults seldom require boosters more often than approximately every 10 years. If an injury occurs which could cause tetanus, it may be necessary to receive a booster toxoid injection to give a patient protection more quickly. For specific information, you should check with your physician concerning current recommendations.

Are reactions ever noted when patients are given tetanus-toxoid?

On occasion, allergic adults in particular may have reactions to tetanus-toxoid. Any individual can develop fever, swelling, or malaise from this vaccine. Some brands, especially in Europe, contain casein or milk in trace amounts which can cause symptoms in milk-sensitive patients. Trace amounts of other substances in vaccines can sometimes cause reactions at the area of an injection or general reactions such as fever.

What is horse serum?

Horse serum is a portion of the blood of horses. If blood coagulates in a test tube, a red clot will form at the bottom, and clear yellow serum will appear above the clot. The serum portion of the blood is the part which contains protection, for example, against tetanus if a horse had been previously immunized with tetanus-toxoid. A horse serum which contains protection is called antitoxin. If it contains tetanus protection, it is called tetanus antitoxin.

Why is tetanus (lockjaw) and diphtheria immunization especially important for allergic individuals?

Anyone who steps on a rusty nail can become ill with tetanus. There are several ways a person can prevent this. If he has had a tetanus toxoid injection in the recent past without any special treatment, he might be able to form protection so rapidly in his body that tetanus would not develop. If he had had tetanus toxoid several years ago, he could receive another toxoid booster and quickly form lockjaw protection in his body. If, however, he had not had an injection of tetanus toxoid for many years or had never had one, he could not form his own protection fast enough to prevent lockjaw, even if he had a booster injection of tetanus toxoid. In such a situation a patient is often given preformed protection against lockjaw in the form of horse serum which contains tetanus antitoxin. (This can be purchased and is obtained from the blood of horses who had received tetanus toxoid.)

If horse antitoxin protection, however, were given to a patient who was allergic to horse serum, the patient would become ill from the horse serum while he was being safeguarded against lockjaw.

Similarly, a person exposed to diphtheria can make his own protection if he has recently had diphtheria toxoid. If he has not, however, he may have to receive diphtheria antitoxin (in horse serum) which would cause a severe immediate reaction in persons allergic to horse serum.

For this reason, careful records should be maintained whenever an allergic individual is immunized so that this information is always readily available.

Is horse serum allergy common?

Many patients who have allergies are sensitive, not only to horse serum, but to all other forms of animal sera. Vaccines made from human serum are less apt to cause allergic symptoms.

Any individual who has an allergy to horse or other serum should wear a name tag or carry a card stating that this is a medical problem (See page 261).

Which medical problems are treated with animal sera?

It is possible for snake or spider bites, rabies, botulism, diphtheria, tetanus, and gas gangrene to be treated with antitoxin prepared from the blood of different types of animals. Allergic individuals could have difficulty if they were sensitive to the animal type of serum used as a source of antitoxin. Horse serum also has been used in kidney and heart transplants.

If an individual is allergic to horse serum, how can he avoid receiving it?

The best method to avoid the need for antitoxin or horse serum would be to receive booster toxoid injections at regular intervals as recommended by your physician. This would mean that an injured person could make his own protection and would not require antitoxin protection produced by some other animal.

What happens if someone allergic to horse serum must receive it?

On occasion, an individual who is allergic to horse serum has to receive this form of protection to help prevent a potentially fatal illness such as lockjaw or tetanus. If a patient cannot form his own protection soon enough, he may have to receive antitoxin protection formed by some other animal to help cope with this disease. If horse serum anti-toxin is given to an individual who is allergic to it, he will be protected against lockjaw but the horse serum can cause an acute allergy medical problem called serum sickness. This could cause a severe reaction in a minute or two. Usually, however, a sensitivity to horse serum caused by an antitoxin occurs 6 to 21 days after the injection. This illness is charac-terized by an itchy welt-like rash, swelling of lymph nodes or glands in the neck, upper legs, or underarms, and swollen joints. Occasionally, a patient will develop weakness or pains in his arms and central nervous system problems.

It is possible by examining a sample of blood to predict whether a patient will develop a serum sickness reaction, but this test requires a special laboratory and facilities which would not be universally avail-able.

CHAPTER SEVENTEEN

Allergies at school

ALLERGIES CAUSED WITHIN SCHOOLS

Can substances found in schools cause allergy?

Yes. Although most children are more allergic to items found in their home and, therefore, have more symptoms during the evening, nights, or weekends, some children have more problems during the school day.

Youngsters in boarding schools or college students who live at school can have problems related to their bedrooms. Student's rooms can be stark and bare, or dusty and cluttered. The bedroom or dormitory should be kept as allergy-free as is sensibly possible. (See page 139). It might be necessary for an allergic child to buy plastic encasings for the mattress and pillows of a roommate.

Children sleeping in dormitories are often required to make their beds at the same time. This creates an atmosphere greatly contaminated with dust, mites, wool, feathers, and moulds which can cause sudden symptoms.

Which school classes can cause allergic symptoms?

There are so many special classes with exposure to unusual substances that it is difficult to discuss all of them. The following, however, could conceivably prove troublesome:

ART CLASS – Dried flowers, vegetation or plant life, use of clay or kilns, contact with wallpaper paste, glue, or various types of cements, glazed paints, tempera or water-colour paint, crayons, cellophane, different types of paper, India or linoleum inks, and marking pencils or pens.

COOKING CLASS – Odour of or eating foods such as eggs, nuts, fish, potatoes or flour.

CLASSROOMS – Any animals with fur or feathers, chalk, cosmetics, perfume, hair spray, after-shaving lotion used by teachers or pupils, printed chemically impregnated or mimeographed paper, stencils, arti-

224

ficial or real flowers, moulds, carpeting or carpet pads, or dust and odours from the heating system.

CHURCH – The odour of perfume, incense, or burning candles. Old churches can smell dusty, musty, and mouldy.

CHEMISTRY – Chemicals or odours from different experiments.

GYMNASTICS – Musty or mouldy locker rooms, dusty gym floors, and gym mats. Outdoor gym classes expose children to pollens and mould spores during the warm months (See page 260) and if the weather is cold, asthmatic episodes can be precipitated.

PRINTING CLASS – Odour of ink or fresh print (flaxseed).

WOODWORKING OR METAL SHOP – Odour of shellacs, lacquers, sawdust, paint-thinners, paints, plastics, smoke, and various types of air pollutants.

Should allergic youths enter competitive sports?

Many excellent athletes have asthma. Asthmatic persons in particular seem to do well when they swim or when they engage in activities which require short bursts of activity such as soccer.

Their performance, however, would be better if an asthma drug could be used *prior to* participation in sports events. It must be remembered that in some sports such as the Olympic games, it is forbidden to take any drugs before competing. A gold medal was taken, unfortunately, from a swimming race winner because he had taken ephedrine before the race. Antihistamines should be avoided because these might interfere with coordination and cause sleepiness.

Should an asthmatic, who wheezes on exertion, take gym class?

In general, the answer is yes. If gym routinely causes breathing difficulty, a child should take his asthma drug ten minutes before class to prevent noticeable symptoms from occurring. If use of a drug prior to gym class, however, does not prevent severe asthma, gym may have to be discontinued, at least temporarily.

At times asthmatic children may begin to wheeze during gym class. If a child who seldom wheezes finds that he is having difficulty breathing, he should immediately discontinue activity and take his asthma drugs. Some children, however, are shy or ashamed of their asthma and refuse to take any treatment. Parents of such children should ask the gym teacher to watch their youngster somewhat more closely so appropriate treatment can be given if necessary.

There are some children who dislike sports and prefer to use their allergies as an excuse so that they do not have to take swimming or gym class. Mature judgement should be used, and a child should not be allowed unjustifiably to use his medical problem as an excuse. This tendency must be strongly discouraged because it could start a most undesirable life-long habit pattern.

Some youths are fond of sports such as soccer but find that this activity causes wheezing. Such individuals can select to play a position which is less strenuous or they may find that a capsule of disodium cromoglycate before the game solves the problem.

Which allergic problems can swimming cause?

Asthmatics seem to tolerate swimming very well. Rarely someone might conceivably have difficulty in heavily chlorinated pools. Chlorine can be irritating and could aggravate eye or nose symptoms. It helps if the eyes are rinsed after swimming by repeatedly opening and closing the eyes in a sink of clean warm water.

Some swimming pool areas smell mouldy or musty and this could precipitate symptoms in persons who have this type of allergy. Algae in water has been known to cause asthma and skin rashes.

Children who have eczema usually tolerate swimming very well even though pools are heavily chlorinated. Strong soaps used when showering after swimming or gym can cause excessive drying of the skin.

Do allergic children have problems from school parties?

Yes. Mothers often bake a cake or something special for an entire class as part of a birthday or special celebration. Food allergic children should always have a suitable substitute in school, provided by their parents, so that they do not accidentally eat eggs, nuts, chocolate, or milk, if these foods cause symptoms.

Will children feel neglected if they cannot play school games, or eat party foods?

They certainly will feel "left out". It is essential that the instructor, teacher, headmaster, and school nurse not only be sympathetic but try to reduce the trauma associated with such a situation. Sometimes unknowing adults ridicule allergic children because they feel their problems are "all emotional". It can only be hoped that parents and physicians might be able to inform school authorities to such a degree that they will be able to understand and help in a meaningful way.

In some schools it is customary for children who have allergies to sit on the sidelines and watch other children play. This is cruel and special provisions should be made for these children so that they can attend a study room or library at that time.

Do school libraries cause allergies?

Often libraries contain books which are dusty and mouldy. Many older books are bound with glue and fish sensitive individuals can have symptoms from the glue or bindings. Allergenic mites also can be found in books. Magazines and new books can cause symptoms in persons allergic to odours of fresh print or certain types of papers.

Can allergic symptoms be caused from a school cafeteria?

Children or teachers with severe food allergies should hesitate to eat a lunch provided in a school cafeteria. In particular, eating eggs, chocolate, milk, fish, nuts, potatoes, wheat, pork products, peas, tomatoes, and certain spices such as cinnamon can cause difficulty. Meals which contain a speck of one of these foods can cause alarming symptoms in some patients.

Symptoms could include itching or swelling of the lips, mouth, tongue, or throat; asthma; eye and nose itching or watering; and digestive problems. A child who innocently shares a nut, chocolate, or pastry with an almond flavouring could conceivably cause grave problems. Refer to page 181 for foods which unexpectedly contain milk, wheat, or eggs.

Does nursery school or kindergarten present special problems?

Young school children frequently sleep directly on the floor during nap time. Children who are allergic to dust should not do this. If it is a rule, these youngsters should sleep on a special mat or towel which is laundered prior to each school day. If the classroom floor is carpeted, it is dusty and can cause allergy.

Children who have allergies frequently wheeze with infections. When any young child first begins school he has less protection against infections than when he is older. The exposure to colds, in particular, is increased. Many children have an excessive number of infections during the first year of school. Asthmatic attacks in allergic children can sometimes be aborted or prevented by treating each infection vigorously when it is first evidenced and starting prophylactic medicines to prevent or treat asthma as soon as possible.

Nursery schools frequently have parties of various types. Exposure to eggs, milk, nuts, and chocolate can cause symptoms in some patients. Fur or feather covered pets may be within the classroom, and are capable of causing symptoms.

Allergic children may have difficulty handling clay, finger paints, putty-like substances, and using glues or cements of various types. Marking pencils frequently cause symptoms.

Should a child or adult who is wheezing go to school?

If someone normally wheezes every day, but the asthma is well-controlled by the use of drugs, he should go to school. If an individual, however, seldom wheezes and begins to have a severe episode during the night, he should not go to school in the morning. If an asthmatic had a difficult night and slept poorly, he should be allowed to rest.

If there is evidence of infection, a physician should be contacted. Whenever anyone wheezes, an effort should be made to determine why the asthma attack occurred on that particular day. Something must be different and only by trying to determine the cause of an episode can insight be secured which might help to prevent future episodes.

Children who are wheezing should never be allowed to attend school merely because *they want to go*. It is most unfortunate that a youngster may have to miss Christmas, a birthday party, the end of term, or some other special occasion in school. If your child is most anxious to attend school, but you know this is unwise, you must *not* allow him to go. If you are unsure, check with your physician and he will help you to make the correct decision. Mothers must not be tempted to send children to school because they have a hair appointment, or something special planned. The youngster should be kept home and a babysitter or neighbour asked to watch the child, if a mother has a previous commitment.

A wheezing child (or adult) should not be allowed to stay home if he is well enough to go to school. Many try to use their asthma as an excuse to avoid examinations or potential unpleasant situations. This must be strongly discouraged.

Must allergic youngsters ride to school?

It depends upon the severity of a youngster's allergies. If the youngster can walk the distance between home and school without difficulty, he does not need to be driven. If the distance is such, however, that symptoms are frequently precipitated, your physician can provide a note requesting school bus transportaion *if this is available*, or parents can arrange to drive the child to school. It frequently helps if medicine is given 20 minutes before it is time to leave for school, and again just before school closes.

Some school buses have noxious fumes which can precipitate chest and nose symptoms of allergies.

During cold weather, cold air can trigger allergic symptoms. This can be diminished by having a person breathe through his nose with his mouth closed or by covering the nose and mouth with a scarf so that the air is warmed before it reaches the lungs. Children who wheeze upon exposure to cold air often require transportation to and from school. Once the allergies are adequately treated and have responded well, this might no longer be required.

Does school cleaning cause allergic symptoms?

It is possible for items used to dust or clean school rooms or to sweep floors to cause allergies. Waxes, polishes, and repairing or maintenance of a school can cause symptoms especially if the items create odours.

Schools which contain carpeting cause allergies even if the carpeting is non-allergic. This is especially true if carpet play or sitting is encouraged. (See page 143).

Which heating system is best for schools?

Most types of heating systems can cause allergies because they produce irritating pollution and diminish the humidity in the atmosphere. Forced hot air heating systems circulate dust. Radiant or electric heat would cause fewer allergies than gas or oil, forced hot air, or hot water systems. (See pages 149 to 151).

Can fire drills precipitate allergic symptoms?

Yes. Some children's allergies are definitely aggravated by fire drills because children may be requested to go outside when they are not properly dressed. Slight chilling seems to trigger wheezing or even infection in some asthmatics. Some children are so sensitive to draughts that sitting near an open window can cause symptoms.

Should you tell the teacher or school nurse about your youngster's allergies?

You cannot give the school too much information. The more they understand your child's problem, the more fully they can cooperate to prevent allergic problems and to give the child adequate care once an allergic problem has arisen. Many schools do not have school nurses and so medically trained personnel may not be available. Because teachers are sometimes ill and substitutes are sent, it is essential that the headmaster be aware of special problems related to your child. The school should always have drugs which are clearly labelled with your child's name and the dose which should be given. The drugs should state why and when they should be given. Your physician can furnish the necessary information. The school should have the telephone number of a child's home, of his mother's and father's place of employment, and of the child's physician so that someone responsible can be contacted should a sudden emergency problem arise. In some countries and in some schools it is against the law for children to carry their own drugs. This means that someone else must be responsible for giving emergency medication, for example, to patients allergic to stinging insects or certain foods.

Can a food allergy cause inattention in school?

This indeed has been reported. For example, some patients are known to have a dull Monday repeatedly, while during the rest of the week they seem to grasp information quickly. This type of reaction is frequently related to a food which is eaten only on Sundays. Children who seem to be bright and alert on certain days and subdued, inattentive, and unable to concentrate on other days can definitely have food allergies. Analysis of foods eaten during the 12 to 24 hours before the "dull" days will often reveal the causative factor. Fish, milk, eggs, chocolate and chicken are common offenders. (See page 163).

What other allergies can interfere with learning?

Nose, eye, or chest allergies which interfere with proper rest can cause chronic fatigue and decrease a child's ability to concentrate while in school. Antihistamines often cause drowsiness.

Ear allergies can cause intermittent hearing loss so that a child might do well on one day, but poorly the next. Chronic formation of fluid behind the eardrums cause a hearing loss over a long period of time which could significantly contribute to a child's poor school performance.

CHAPTER EIGHTEEN

Holiday travel and camping

Should allergic patients take holidays in the country?

It depends entirely upon a person's allergies. If an individual has mild pollen or mould spore problems, camping may cause little difficulty. If the proper drugs are taken prior to or during a stay in the country, symptoms should be readily controlled. If the patient has major difficulty during the warm months, excess exposure to pollens or moulds, may cause extreme symptoms.

Most pollen-sensitive patients who have received allergy extract treatment seem to do well when they visit the countryside. In general, persons who have allergies should act as much as possible as persons who don't have allergies.

Are there special summer holiday areas in Europe for asthmatics?

These may be high up in the mountains, at special spas, or at the seaside. Many asthmatic children go home during the summer holiday, but in France, they will go anytime during the summer to take the cure at such places at La Bourboule. Adults go to Le Mont Dore. One country cannot be compared with another.

When is the "best time" to holiday?

Parents should try to select a time when the allergic person has the least amount of symptoms. On page 260 are found pollen calendars for many areas of the world. From examining these, it should be possible to determine when and where pollens are evident and it might be possible to select a time and place where less difficulty should arise.

What sleeping accomodations are best when one's on holiday?

Highly allergic persons should try to sleep in hotel rooms which are not dusty, or musty. Rooms which smell mouldy or of stagnant smoke should be avoided. Allergic patients should try to carry their own pillows, a plastic mattress cover, and a room air-purifier. The purifier can be used constantly in the room to help eliminate airborne allergenic substances. Woollen blankets should be sandwiched in the middle of the bedding so they are not pulled directly under a patient's nose during sleep. Feather comforters cannot be used. Caravan travel is fine providing they are kept very clean. Caravans often smell stale or mouldy after long periods of not being used. They must be scrubbed thoroughly and aired prior to use. Inside dust is more likely to cause allergies than outside dirt.

Which factors related to camplife cause allergic symptoms?
    1.   HIKING AND NATURE STUDY – This can conceivably cause difficulties because individuals could be exposed to plant pollen, leather products, fur, or other items which could cause allergic symptoms. Prophylactically, antihistamines or drugs used to treat asthma can be taken prior to exposure and if symptoms do not become extreme, it is possible to continue engaging in the usual camp activities.
    2.   CAMPFIRES – Allergic patients should always sit in such a way that the smoke from the campfire does not blow towards them. Irritation from campfire (or tobacco) smoke can trigger eye, nose, and chest symptoms.
    3.   SLEEPING – Dusty cabins, cottages or mouldy tents must be avoided. Sweeping and cleaning such accommodations could cause symptoms. Sleeping bags must never be filled with down, but rather with a synthetic fibre and must be laundered prior to use. If they were damp when they were stored, they could be mouldy. Patients must not sleep on dusty mattresses unless they are *covered entirely* with clean plastic and they must not sleep on straw filled mats. If possible, allergic persons should carry their own synthetic pillows and clean freshly laundered bedding. Room air-purifiers could be used only in cabins or caravans which had electricity.
    4.   FOODS – Persons with major food allergies (such as to eggs, milk, or wheat) should carry an adequate supply of foods which they can tolerate when they camp. If there is a camp cook, the allergic problems should be discussed in detail. It is possible for a major food allergy to present an unreasonable inconvenience for all concerned. Patients unfamiliar with food allergies seldom realize that the mere smell or a speck of a food could cause immediate alarming reaction for some patients.
    5.   ANIMALS – Many campsites have animals. Avoidance is stressed if a patient has symptoms even though he has been premedicated prior to exposure. If an individual, however, finds that he can ride a horse providing that he does not enter the stable or attempt to brush the animal, then he should ride as much as he likes providing he continues to feel well. He may have to bathe and change his clothing immediately after riding.

6.   SPORTS ACTIVITIES – Many summer camps have swimming and other sports facilities. In general, asthmatic children should take asthma drugs prior to engaging in this activity to prevent or diminish wheezing. If they begin to wheeze badly, they should stop play and not resume the activity until they're feeling better. If they continually have difficulty when they attempt to exercise, they should try to occupy themselves with some other activity.

Antihistamines should not be taken prior to sports because they can cause drowsiness and poor co-ordination. Antihistamines, however, can be taken as soon as the activity is completed if nose symptoms are a problem.

If the patient's eyes seem to be irritated from chlorine used in pools, it is helpful if the eyes are bathed with clear water after swimming. An antihistamine might be helpful. Nose and eye symptoms of allergies are less if a face mask is worn over the eyes and nose. This allows underwater activity without irritation of the eyes and nose.

Diving and underwater swimming should be discouraged for anyone who has had recurrent ear problems caused by the accumulation of fluid behind the eardrum.

Some patients are allergic to cold water. Contact can cause welts (nettle rash) or wheezing. Persons who have this type of physical allergy should be extremely careful not to jump into a pool or stream unless they are certain that the water is warm. If they were exposed to a large amount of cold water suddenly, it is possible for chemicals to be released within their body which could cause fainting. This could cause a very dangerous situation in a swimming pool.

Algae in swimming pools and lakes have been reported to cause asthma and skin rashes. This can successfully be treated with allergy extract injections.

Most asthmatics tend to be worse if they are chilled, exhausted, or exercise in excess. For this reason, asthmatics should be warned to attempt to carry out sports activity in moderation so that they will remain well enough to participate in other camp programmes. Those who have found disodium cromoglycate (INTAL) effective in preventing asthma should be certain to inhale this BEFORE exercise. It will not help if it is used afterwards.

Are special considerations necessary when allergic persons travel?

Travel often precipitates allergic symptoms in patients who may have been well for some time. The following considerations might help prevent allergies from ruining a holiday.

1.   DRUGS – Patients on holiday must always carry an adequate supply of well-labelled drugs. Each drug should clearly state how often

and why it should be taken. If potential problems are anticipated, allergic emergencies can often be aborted or prevented. If exposure to highly allergenic factors is unavoidable, a drug such as disodium cromoglycate (Intal) should be used PRIOR to exposure. Be certain to carry the phone number of your physician so he can be called if this is necessary. If emergencies arise which cannot be controlled, go to the nearest hospital or seek the help of a nearby physician. If a patient has a severe food allergy or a stinging insect problem, adrenaline or an aerosol should be available for immediate use because such problems could prove critical before trained medical help could be secured.

Patients who travel should be certain always to wear a name tag stating their exact food, drug, or type of allergy. They should also have their tetanus-toxoid immunization up to date prior to leaving their home. See page 261.

2.   INFECTION – Many asthmatics wheeze badly with most infections. If both antibiotics and asthma medicines are given immediately, it is often possible to abort and easily control the attacks. When travelling, it is not always easy to secure medical help. Some patients should carry drugs to treat infections such as a sore throat or earache which can be used until proper medical care is possible. Care should be taken so that asthma is not allowed to continue for several days without receiving medical help.

3.   FOODS – Families who travel may be able to carry or purchase much of their food supply so that food allergies may not be a problem. It is often necessary, however, to eat at restaurants and this could be dangerous for persons with major food allergies. Adults or parents of allergic children must be knowledgeable about potential hidden sources of foods which often cause allergy.

4.   RELATIVES AND FRIENDS – Many problems arise when visiting relatives and friends because of dust and pets. Allergic patients often begin to wheeze and are reluctant to return home or stay at a motel because they do not want to offend their hosts. The tendency is to try to weather the storm by remaining in an allergenic atmosphere. Quite often the patient becomes progressively more and more ill. The only sensible solution is either to avoid the problem entirely by initially staying at a motel or returning home sooner than anticipated. Relatives will accept a good reason if you are reluctant to give the real reason for your early departure.

5.   SMOKING – If anyone smokes tobacco in a car while a family is travelling, it can aggravate asthma or nose and eye symptoms of allergies. For the sake of all, this should not be allowed.

6.   MISCELLANEOUS FACTORS – The use of insect repellent sprays, candles, or outside cookers can cause irritating which trigger allergic symptoms. Fatigue, chilling, and excitement should be avoided

if possible. The route and time for travelling should be carefully studied to avoid passing through or staying in places which have a high pollen count of the type to which you are allergic.

Should a patient receive an allergy-extract while travelling?

It may not be necessary for a patient to receive an injection of extract while he's on holiday if he received an extra treatment before his travels began and will return home before he is due for his next treatment. Discuss what is best for you with your physician.

Treatments can often be obtained from hospital physicians or other doctors during travel. In countries with free medical health programmes such as Great Britain, injection treatments would *not* be given in clinics, unless the person came from a country which had a similar health programme and extended reciprocity. Allergy physicians in private practice would give allergy injection therapy when needed.

Could a physician refuse to give an allergy-extract treatment?

Many physicians would be reluctant to give anyone an allergy-extract treatment if the patient could not provide adequate information. The following would be essential and necessary:

1. The extract should be well-labelled and state the name of the patient and a description of the contents. For example, it should state grass, weed, tree, or allergy extract. The label should also note the strength and the expiration date (e.d.) of the medicine. A special slip should instruct the doctor concerning the dose and date by which treatment must be administered. Examples of properly labelled extracts are given below.

Mary Jones	Tom White
Weed Extract	Dust Extract
10,000 p.n.u.	1:10
dose due by 24/Nov./1974*	dose due by 24/Nov./1974*
0.5 cc 10,000 p.n.u.	0.7 cc. 1:10
e.d. Dec., 1974	e.d. Dec., 1974

All of the above information and instructions can be obtained from your regular physician, but you should check to be certain that *all* of the above information is included. Depend only upon yourself to do this, because if any of the information is lacking and the extract dosage is

---

e.d. = expiration date for allergy extract

* Dates can be expressed differently depending upon the country in which you live. In Canada, the month is put first, in Great Britain, it is put second. This can cause confusion for foreign physicians.

overdue, it will create more difficulties when the next dosage of extract is finally given.

The patient must be certain to return the extract *with a slip* stating the date and dose which he received while on holiday. These details are essential and necessary so that there will be no problem when the next dosage of extract is administered *after* the patient has returned home.

Do special precautions need to be taken to refrigerate an allergy extract while travelling?

No. Allergy extracts are often mailed to distant places which may require several days. It should not cause any difficulty, therefore, if a new sterile extract were not refrigerated for a few days. If the holiday will last for many days, keep the extract refrigerated but not frozen, as much of the time as possible.

How can you find out who are allergists in foreign countries?

Check with your allergist prior to travelling.

CHAPTER NINETEEN

Allergies related to celebrations

What allergic problems arise in relation to Easter?
Most symptoms are caused by eating chocolate, nuts (nut flavouring in chocolate), and eggs. Pink, white, or yellow chocolate is as allergenic as brown chocolate. Certain brands of chocolate may cause allergic symptoms while others will not. Chocolate-sensitive patients sometimes can substitute "chocolate" made from soybeans. This often smells but does not taste like chocolate. Soybean chocolate could cause difficulty in peanut-sensitive patients.

Some patients can eat hard-boiled eggs, but would have difficulty with less well-cooked eggs.

The dyes, spices, and flavouring of certain sweets can cause allergic symptoms. Licorice is a legume and can cause difficulty in soybean or peanut sensitive patients.

Are there special problems related to Christmas?

CHRISTMAS TREES

Some patients are allergic to evergreen trees. The exact reason is unclear. The odour of pine or moulds on the trees might be possible factors. Some people have difficulty as they approach a stand of Christmas trees. Others have difficulty from the moment the tree is set up in their home until it is removed. Many persons develop an itchy contact-type rash from touching evergreens. Some patients have been found to be sensitive to one type of evergreen but not to others. For example, they could be allergic to firs but not to spruces. Decorations with branches or the use of pine sprays, soaps, bath oils, incense, or scented candles can cause symptoms. Exposure to evergreens can be unavoidable because of trees in stores, classrooms, or home of friends. Appropriate drugs (i.e. Intal for asthmatics) given prior to unavoidable exposure is sometimes helpful. If a person is sensitive, it often helps if an artificial tree is used. These, however, can be sprayed with dyes or have an offensive odour capable of causing symptoms.

CHRISTMAS DECORATIONS

A second problem is related to home decorations. These are frequently saved from year to year and stored in dusty or even musty or mouldy areas. Bringing decorations from a storage area, opening the boxes, and helping to place them about the house can cause symptoms. Stuffed decorations often acquire an "old" odour which can cause symptoms.

CHRISTMAS FOODS

The special foods which are eaten during the Christmas holidays can cause allergies. For example, the odour of a dish of nuts can cause difficulty. If a peanut-allergic person selects walnuts from a dish of mixed nuts, it is possible that there might be enough peanut on the walnut to cause immediate symptoms. Patients who are allergic to eggs sometimes forget and drink eggnogs during the holidays.

CHRISTMAS EXCITEMENT

Children in particular tend to become fatigued by staying up too late and this combined with the great excitement which surrounds the holiday can seem to cause asthma. It is helpful if drugs to prevent or treat asthma are given the day before Christmas as well as during the entire holiday.

If an individual goes carolling, the cold air can cause wheezing unless the mouth is covered with a scarf and breathing is through the nose, not the mouth. This, however, would interfere with singing. Slow walks in the cold outdoors, especially when combined with mouth breathing can cause sudden asthma. Prophylactic drugs should be given to help prevent this from occurring.

NEW YEAR'S EVE

On this gala occasion, many persons drink alcohol, particularly champagne or fermented beverages which contain moulds or yeasts. These can cause allergies in some individuals. See page 147. Herring could cause symptoms in fish-sensitive patients.

Do birthday parties cause allergies?
They certainly do. Birthday foods include cake, which can contain milk, wheat, nuts, nut flavouring, chocolate, eggs, and certain dyes. All of these cause symptoms in some individuals. Eggwhite cake frosting and birthday candles can also be a factor. Cinnamon-glazed apples cause symptoms. This special occasion is associated with excitement and fatigue so drugs to prevent or treat allergy should be started the day before the birthday and continued until the celebration is over.

What activities in relation to Jewish holidays cause allergies?
CHANUKAH – Holiday decorations used on this day are stored and used year after year. These can become dusty, musty, and smell "old." Burning candles can also cause symptoms.

Foods eaten on this day can cause symptoms because they may contain nuts, wheat, eggs (in potato pancakes), or onions.
PASSOVER – The most common food eaten at this time is matzah. Traditionally, this is composed of wheat, but various flavourings, as well as eggs, can cause symptoms. Nuts, chicken, wine, and apples (insect spray if they are not washed adequately) could be factors.
PURIM – Hamantashen made with eggs, flour, cooking oil and sometimes filled with prunes or poppy seed is eaten on this day.
ROSH HASHANAH – Common foods causing problems would include gefilte fish, nuts, chicken, spices, eggs, and wine (could be a problem for mould or yeast sensitive patients).
YOM KIPPUR – At this time chicken and kreplach which contains eggs, wheat, and spices are frequently eaten. After fasting, fish of different types are eaten including gefilte fish, pickled herring with spices, lox (salmon), and tuna fish. Other holiday foods are challah (yeast and eggs) and farfel which contains flour and eggs.

Which Mohammedan feast foods cause allergies?
On feast days, both children and adults may be encouraged to eat sweet meals containing honey, nuts, milk, wheat, etc., some of which, after a period of not eating, could cause symptoms.

Which Chinese holiday foods could cause allergy?
The Chinese use flavouring such as sodium glutamate in their soups and sauces which can cause acute allergic-like reactions in some sensitive individuals. Fish, nuts, and soy sauce are also used in their special preparations.

APPENDIX I

Possible allergenic substances

BUCKWHEAT*

pancake flours or Jewish Kasha
buckwheat grits or cereal is often used to line pans used to bake rye or
   pumpernickel bread. It prevents burning.

CORN*

SMELL

popping corn
boiling corn on cob
certain body powders

certain bath powders
ironing certain starched clothes

TASTE

corn flakes
corn flour
corn meal
corn oil (Mazola)
cornstarch
corn sugars
corn syrups (Karo)

grits
hominy
popped corn
fresh corn
canned or frozen corn
succotash

*From Theron Randolph, *Human Ecology and Susceptibility to the Chemical Environment*, 1967, Charles C Thomas, Publisher, Springfield, Illinois. Used by permission.

CORN IN SOME FORM

adhesives: envelopes, stickers,
    stamps, tapes
aspirin
bacon
baking mixes
baking powders
beer
beverages
bologna
bourbon
breads or pastries
candy
catsup
Cheerios
chewing gum
chili
chop suey
coffee (instant)
confectioner's sugar
custards
dates
deep-fat frying oils
diluents for gelatin capsules,
   lozenges, ointments, suppositories, tablets
flour, bleached
fried food
Fritos
frostings
fruit juices, especially grape juice
fruits
graham crackers
gravies
grits
ham
hominy
ice-cream

jams
jellies
liquor (bourbon)
lunchmeat
margarine – some types
milk in paper cartons
monosodium glutamate
oleomargarine
pablum
paper containers (when wet)
peanut butter
pies, creamed
plastic food wrappers
Post Toasties
powdered sugar
puddings
salad dressing
salt
sandwich spreads
sauces for gravy, fish, meats,
   sundaes
sausages
sherbets
Similac
soups
soy-bean milks
teas (instant)
toothpastes or powders
tortillas
vegetables, especially beets,
   canned peas, and string
   beans
vinegar
vitamins
wieners
yeasts
Zest

COTTONSEED

candy, especially chocolate
cosmetics
cotton linters in furniture
cottonseed oil (Cooking oils, i.e.,
   Wesson, are believed to be
   nonallergenic.)

doughnuts
feed for cattle or poultry
fertilizer
fish
mayonnaise
miner's lamp oil

oleomargarines such as Nucoa,
    Good Luck
potato chips
salad dressing
sardines may be in cottonseed oil
shortenings such as Crisco
some medicines such as
    camphorated oil

FLAXSEED SOURCES

These include chair mats, cough remedies, depilatories, dust from linoleum, feed for animals, fiber board, flaxseed tea, insulating material, linen cloth, linseed-oil paints and varnishes, painter's and lithographic inks, plaster, Roman meal bread, straw hats, stuffing for furniture, wave-set lotions, wet newsprint (boys with this sensitivity should not be newsboys or should wear gloves when delivering papers)

GINGER

ginger ale, ginger beer, preserves, cookies or cake

GUMS (VEGETABLE)

Indian, Karaya, or Tragacanth are binders used to hold together tablet forms of medicine or to thicken foods or liquids, such as:

cake icing (commercially prepared)
cheeses (cream and others)
chewing gum
diabetic foods
denture adhesives
emulsified mineral oils
face powders
gelatins
gumdrop candy or jelly beans
ice-cream fillers
laxatives
lotions (hand and face)
lozenges
marshmallows
mouthwash
mustard
pie fillings
potato salad
rouge
salad dressing
soft-centered candy
toothpastes or powders
wave-set lotion
wheat cakes or flour
whipped cream
white sauces

HAIR

COW HAIR

blankets
brushes
certain carpets
"Ozite" rug pads (waffle-iron
    weave)
plaster
roofing felt for covering boilers or
    for insulation
rope
sofas and some cushions
stables or cows

GOAT HAIR

artificial furs
blankets
carpets
cashmere clothing
felt hats
goats

mohair items—sweaters, suits, coats
mops
oriental rugs
plaster
ropes
water-proofing fabrics

HOG HAIR

brushes
hogs
pads for rugs

HORSEHAIR

certain hats
clothing exposed to horsehair
cushions
plasters
ropes

stables and horses
some brushes
some chairs
some mattresses
wigs

RABBIT FUR OR HAIR

angora
coat trimming, muffs, rabbit's
    feet
felt hats

felt in sounding hammers of pianos
pillows, quilts, sweaters
rabbits or rabbit hutches

PYRETHRUM

Patients allergic to this substance frequently are also sensitive to ragweed or to plants in the chrysanthemum family because of a close botanical relationship. Florists or children frequently exposed to many flowers often become allergic to it. Pyrethrum is also found in some insecticides (both spray or powder), some plant sprays, and some ointments or medicines used to treat skin parasites.

Children who have symptoms when exposed to insect sprays can sometimes tolerate a liquid (such as OFF) applied directly to the clothing.

KAPOK

This is a fiber of the silk-cotton tree found in Asia. It is silky and white and resembles dried milkweed-pod filling. It is used mainly to stuff toys, pillows, mattresses, comforters, and in upholstery and life jackets.

SOYBEAN PRODUCTS (both meal and oil)*

FOOD PRODUCTS

baked goods
candy, caramels, hard candy,
    nut candy
certain cereals, grits
certain diet foods
Chinese foods with soy sprouts
cooking oils
Crisco or Spry
ice cream
LaChoy sauce
lecithin, sometimes derived from
    soybean
margarine
mayonnaise
medicinal oil
milk substitutes as Sobee, Neo-
    Mull-Soy, Soyalac, Valectin
pork sausage, wieners, lunch meats
seasoning powders
soups
soy nuts
wine or in brewing of beer
Worcestershire sauce

INDUSTRIAL USES

Factories utilizing soy products can contaminate the air with enough of this substance to cause allergies in some very sensitive persons.

animal food
artificial wool
caking compound
candles
celluloid
cosmetics
disinfectants
electrical insulation
emulsifier
enamels
fertilizer
fire-fighting foam
fuel
glue and adhesives
glycerin
insecticides
leather dressing
lighting
linoleum
oil cloth
paints
painting ink
plastics
rubber substitutes
soaps
synthetic resins
textile dressing
varnishes
waterproofing
whipping powder

*From Joseph H. Fries, "Studies on the Allergenicity of Soybean," *Annals of Allergy*, 29:1, January, 1971. Used by permission of the author and publisher.

APPENDIX II

Food and diet aids

COMMON RELATED FOODS AND GRAINS

If there are obvious symptoms from one food in a group, it is possible the others might also cause difficulty.

apple, pear, quince
banana (plantain)
filbert, hazelnut, wintergreen
buckwheat, rhubarb
cashew, pistachio, mango
grapefruit, kumquat, lemon, lime, orange, tangerine
chocolate, cola
mushroom, yeast
beets, spinach, and the weed lamb's quarters
cantaloupe, cucumber, pumpkin, squash, gherkin, melon
corn, barley, oats, rice, rye, wheat, sugar cane
blueberry, cranberry, huckleberry
avocado, bayleaf, cinnamon, sassafras
asparagus, chive, garlic, leek, onion, sarsaparilla, shallot
marshmallow, okra, cottonseed
lavender, oregano, peppermint, spearmint, sage, savory, thyme
broccoli, brussels sprouts, cabbage, mustard, radish, turnip, collards,
    cress, horseradish
allspice, clove
green or red pepper (cayenne), paprika, eggplant, white potato, tomato
coconut, date
anise, caraway seed, carrot, celery, dill, fennel, parsley, parsnip
acacia, lentils, peas, chick peas, beans (kidney, navy, pinto, string),
    licorice, soybeans, peanuts
almond, apricot, cherry, peach, plum
raspberry, blackberry, boysenberry, strawberry, loganberry

artichoke, burdock, chicory, dandelion, endive, lettuce, tarragon
black walnut, butternut, English walnut, hickory nut, pecan

ANIMAL FOODS

Mollusks: clams, oysters, scallops
Crustaceans: crabs, shrimp, lobster, crayfish
"Red fish": salmon, tuna, trout
"White fish": most other fish

   If your child is sensitive to fish, he should avoid licking stamps, envelopes, using Lepage's glue, or taking cod-liver oil tablets or liquid (see pp. 184-185). Fish glue is also found in book bindings, used in furniture manufacture, in rug sizing, shipping tapes, and straw hats.

POSSIBLE COMMON FOOD SOURCES OF
MILK, WHEAT, AND EGGS

Milk[a]

Wheat

Eggs

au gratin foods

baked goods[b,c]

butter

candy[b]

casein or caseinate

cheese

chocolate

cottage cheese

creamed or
    scalloped foods

curds

custard

gravy

ice cream

malted milk

margarine[d]

milk sherbet

pudding

salad dressing

soups[b]

waffle and biscuit
    mixes

whey

white sauces

wieners or bologna[b]

skim milk

baked goods

biscuits

breads[e,f] (including

rye, rice, etc.)

bread crumbs

breakfast cereals[b]

buns

candy[b]

cereals

coffee substitutes[b]

crackers

cracker meal

doughnuts

dumplings

gravy

ice-cream cones

macaroni, etc.

macaroons

malt (beer)

noodles

pancakes

piecrusts

pretzels

rolls

salad dressing

sauces for vegetable
    or meat

soups (bisques or
    chowders)

spaghetti

stuffing

Swiss steak

wieners or bologna

waffles

albumin

baked goods[f]

Bavarian creams

bread crumbs

breaded foods

candy[b]

coffee[b]

creamed foods

croquettes

crusts – if shiny
    (bread, etc.)

custards

egg white or
    powdered or
    dried egg

French ice cream

French toast

fritters

frostings

mayonnaise

meat loaf

meringue

noodles

pie filling

root beer[b]

salad dressing

sauces
    (Hollandaise)

sausage

soups[b]

waffles

Note: Read all food labels very carefully.

[a]Kosher foods that contain neither milk nor meat are labelled "parve"and should not contain caseinate.

[b]Some, not all.

[c]Italian bread is *often* milk-free.

[d]Kosher margarine is acceptable.

[e]Make unseasoned Ry-Krisp sandwiches, all bread contains wheat.

[f]When baking, substitute ½ teaspoon baking powder for each egg omitted from the recipe. For source of egg-free baking powder, see page 281.

[g]Milk of magnesia has no milk in it.

Thanks are due to Dr. Jerome Glaser of Rochester, N.Y., for much of the information in this list.

'Good' Room

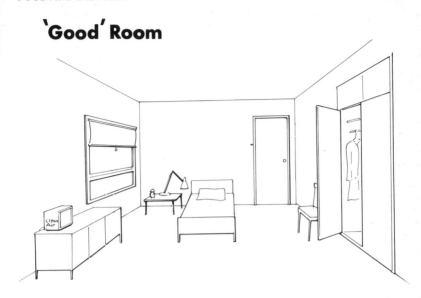

'Bad' Room

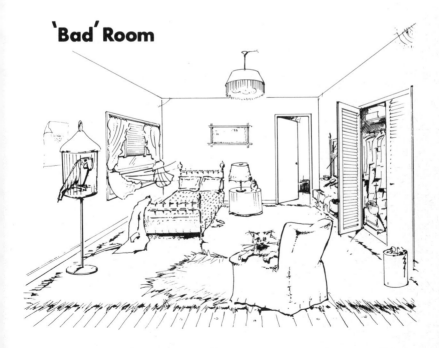

RECIPES FOR SAMPLE DIET OMITTING MILK, EGGS, FISH, NUTS AND FRUITS CONTAINING PIPS

YOU CAN EAT

Beef, mutton, lamb, mince, tongue.
Green vegetables, lettuce, carrots, potatoes, sweetcorn.
Apples, pears, bananas, rhubarb, pineapple.
Butter-free margarine, corn oil (for cooking).
Bread, pastry, cakes, biscuits, (avoid cream cakes and ones with egg in them).
Sugar, syrup.
Tea and instant coffee.
Rice and cornflour.
Porridge.
Non-citrus fruit juices.
'Coffee-mate' instead of milk.

YOU MUST NOT EAT

Milk-ordinary, powdered or tinned. Butter, Cream, Yoghurt etc.
Egg, custard, salad cream, mayonnaise, chicken.
Nuts and pips, tomatoes, tomato sauce, blackcurrants, blackcurrant juice, gooseberries, strawberries, raspberries, oranges, and other citrus fruits, fruit juices and squashes, melons, cucumber, marrow, peas, beans, peanuts.
Marmalade, jam, chocolate, chocolate drinks, fruit sweets, lollies, marzipan, macaroons.
Spices and curry, Chinese and Indian dishes.
Marmite, Oxo, Bovril, gravy-browning, packet soups.
Fish.
Cheese.
Onions, garlic.
Pork, bacon, ham, brawn, all liver, all sausages and canned meat.
Shellfish.
Fizzy drinks.
Beers, ales, stout, lagers, wines, sherry.
Chewing-gum.

BREAKFASTS

Cornflakes or Shreddies with fruit syrup.
Porridge made with water and served with either brown sugar or golden syrup.
Tinned pears, pineapple, stewed apples, fried bananas.
Very thinly sliced silverside topside.
Grilled sausage and pineapple.
Toast or bread with brown or white sugar, treacle, pineapple or apricot jam.
Weetabix spread with plenty of margarine and syrup.

SOUPS

OXTAIL SOUP

1 lb. oxtail
2 pts. water
1 oz. margarine or dripping
Salt and pepper
8 oz. celery, turnip and carrot
1½ oz. flour

Separate the tail into joints. Cover with cold water. Wipe joints. Fry in melted margarine. Add stock and prepared vegetables and seasoning. Bring to the boil and simmer for 3 to 4 hours. Strain and remove meat from the bones and cut into pieces. Blend flour with cold water. Add to the soup together with meat and vegetables. Bring to boil, skim, serve very hot.

VEGETABLE SOUP

1 lb. carrots
1 lb. celery
1 lb. turnip
2 pts. water or oxtail soup
1 oz. margarine
1 tbs. flour
Salt and pepper

Melt margarine. Cut vegetables into small pieces. Sauté in the margarine until soft. Add flour and cook for 5 mins. Add water or stock slowly and simmer for ½-1 hr. Sieve or liquidize soup. Reheat. Add salt and pepper. If the vegetables have been cut very small, the soup will not need sieving.

ARTICHOKE SOUP

2 lbs. artichokes
1 pt. water or oxtail stock
2 oz. margarine or 3 tbs. corn oil
1 oz. flour
Salt and pepper

Wash and peel artichokes. Put peeled artichokes in water until all are finished. Melt margarine. Slice the artichokes into melted margarine/oil. Add salt and pepper. Turn down heat and put lid on saucepan. Sweat artichokes until they are transparent, 10/15 mins. Mash until potato-like. Add the flour and cook for three minutes. Take saucepan off heat. Add water or oxtail. Put saucepan back on heat and stir until soup boils.

APPLE SOUP

2 lbs. apples
1 teacup water
½ pt. oxtail stock
1 oz. cornflour
1 glass cider dry or sweet

Wash apples, peel and core, slice thinly. Put apples into saucepan. Add 1 teacup water and boil very fast with lid until apples disintegrate. Put cornflour in a bowl, add a little oxtail, mix to a smooth paste. Add rest of oxtail to paste. Add oxtail/cornflour liquid to apple. Salt and pepper. Put saucepan back on heat and stir until soup thickens slightly. Add cider and little sugar if necessary.

MEATS

BEEF AND VEGETABLE OLIVES

4 large thin slices of stewing beef
1 lb. carrots
½-1 pt. water/oxtail stock
1 small tin sweet corn
For the stuffing:
1 breakfast cup of breadcrumbs
2 level tablespoons shredded suet
1 tbs. chopped parsley
1 tbs. mint
Water

Soften carrots and mushrooms in a little fat and add to oxtail. Mix all ingredients for stuffing together. Spread on the thin slices of meat. Roll these firmly and tie with pieces of cotton. Fry for a few minutes in hot fat. Put in a casserole and pour over the oxtail and vegetables. Cover with a lid and cook in a slow oven for 2 hours. Garnish with parsley and serve with mashed potatoes.

STEAK AND MACARONI CASSEROLE

3 oz. quick cooking macaroni
1 lb. stewing steak
1 pt. oxtail stock, water or cider
1½ oz. corn oil
1½ oz. flour
1 celery stalk

Cut meat into neat pieces. Prepare celery and cut up. Melt oil and fry meat gently. Remove meat and add flour and cook until brown. Add stock gradually and bring to the boil, stir until smooth. Put in meat and celery. Cover pan and cook gently for 2-2½ hrs.* 10 mins. before serving, add uncooked macaroni. Boil fairly quickly to cook macaroni. *An asbestos mat may be needed under the pan to ensure that it cooks slowly.

LAMB CASSEROLE

2½ lbs. middle neck of lamb
1 large tin sweet corn
3 sticks of celery
1½ pts. of cider or water
1 lb. carrots

Fry lamb on both sides lightly. Add celery and carrots and fry until soft. Put lamb, celery, carrots and sweet corn and cider into casserole. Cook in a moderate oven for 2-2½ hrs.

MINCED BALLS

1 lb. Mince
4 oz. beef sausage meat
2 oz. soft breadcrumbs
2 tbs. chopped parsley
2 tbs. minced raw carrot
1 tbs. minced raw celery
1 pt. beef stock or water
1 oz. cornflour
Golden breadcrumbs

Mix the meat, crumbs, salt and pepper, vegetables and sufficient stock or water to moisten. Form into balls about egg size, and roll in golden breadcrumbs. Melt 1 oz. margarine and fry meat balls quickly in hot fat. Put meat balls in a casserole dish. Add stock or water and seasoning and cook gently for 1-1½ hrs. Put cornflour in small bowl, add a little water and mix to a paste. Add a cupful of hot liquid from the casserole to the cornflour, stirring constantly. Add the thickened gravy to casserole and stir carefully to blend. Serve with carrots and boiled potatoes.

MINCED BEEF

1 oz. flour
½ pt. stock or water
1 lb. minced beef
1 tbs. oil
1 stick celery
1 small tin sweet corn or ½ lb. mushrooms or mushroom stalks

Soften celery and mushrooms in a little oil. Add mince to vegetables and fry lightly. Add flour and stir in thoroughly. Cook for 2 mins. Add stock slowly mixing thoroughly. Add salt and pepper and sweet corn. Cook on very low heat or on asbestos mat for 30 mins.

CORNISH PASTIES

4 oz. flour ⎫
2 oz. marg ⎬ *for shortcrust pastry*
3 oz. cooked meat
1 tbs. cooked diced potato
1 dsp. minced celery and carrot

Chop or mince meat finely. Mix with potato and vegetables. Season. Moisten with a little stock or gravy if very dry. Divide pastry into three equal pieces and roll out thinly into slightly oval shapes. Place a portion of mixture on each piece. Damp edges and fold over. Stand pasties on baking tray with the join in the pastry at the top. Flute edges with finger and thumb. Bake in a hot oven for 20 mins. 400°F or reg 6. Raw vegetables and meat may be used. Pasties should then be cooked for ¾ hr. Reduce heat to 325°F or Reg 4 after 10 mins.

RISOTTO

12 oz. patna rice
2 sticks celery
1 tin sweet corn
8 oz. mushrooms
2 pts. beef stock
2 oz. margarine
2 oz. cold meat (silverside, remains of Sunday joint)

Chop celery finely and fry lightly in 1 oz. marg. until soft. Wash and slice mushrooms, fry gently for 5 mins. Add rice and cover with boiling stock, season and cook gently for about 25 mins. Remove from heat and add drained sweet corn and finely chopped parsley and serve.

LAMB KEBABS

6 lamb cutlets
Salt and pepper
½ oz. margarine or 1 tbs. oil
8 oz. mushrooms
1 small tin pineapple cubes
½ lb. beef sausages

Cut each cutlet into three pieces. Brush with oil. Skewer meat, mushrooms, pineapple and sausage alternately. Sprinkle with salt and pepper. Grill gently Reg 4 turning frequently for about 20 mins. Serve with rice and green salad.

STEAK PIE

½ lb. flour for rough pastry
1 lb. stewing steak
1 tbs. seasoned flour
¼ pt. water or stock

See recipe book for rough puff pastry. Cut meat into neat cubes, dip in seasoned flour. Pack into 1 pt. pie dish, cover pie with pastry. Put pie in a hot oven 400°F or Reg 6. When set and browning, reduce heat to 350°F/Reg 4 until pie cooked. 1½ hrs.

GRILLED LAMB CHOPS WITH BRAISED PINEAPPLE

4 lamb chops
1 tin pineapple rings

Grill chops under moderate grill (Reg 4-5) for 16-20 mins. Turn chops after 10 mins. Take 1 pineapple ring to each chop. Brush both sides with oil. Place under grill with the chops for the last 5 mins.

General Points

A very good casserole can be made on the top of the oven using either a double saucepan or a thick bottomed saucepan resting on two asbestos mats.

When using a double saucepan, bring the casserole to the boil before placing it on to the bottom pan, which should be ½ full of boiling water, Allow 2-3 hours and stir frequently. This method is much more economical than using the whole oven for one dish.

Fruit crumbles, flapjacks, etc. can be cooked at the same time as a casserole, at the temp. recommended for the casserole so long as they are as high as possible in the oven.

Supermarkets' own brand of sausages seem to be the only all beef ones.

DESSERTS

BANANA CUSTARD

Custard may be made with water instead of milk and is quite acceptable. The addition of a little vanilla essence improves the flavour. Slice the bananas into the custard just before serving.

BANANA SURPRISE

Thick slices of French bread
Bananas
Banana butter
Make a hole in the middle of each piece of bread. Spread with banana butter. Put a piece of banana into slice of bread.

BANANA BUTTER

2 oz. margarine
1 large banana
Cream the margarine in a basin and gradually mash the banana into this.

BAKED BANANA

4 firm bananas
2-3 oz. Barbados sugar
1½ oz. Margarine
Peel bananas and lay them in a fireproof dish. Sprinkle lavishly with sugar. Dot with small pieces of margarine. Bake in a fairly hot oven for about 20 mins. till the bananas are soft but not squashy.

CRUMBLE

4 oz. flour
3 oz. margarine
1 oz. brown sugar
Rub fat into the flour until like fine breadcrumbs. Add the sugar. Sprinkle over cooked fruit. Cook in a moderately hot oven for 30 mins. 375°F/Reg 5. Serve with custard or fruit sauce made with some of the water used to cook the fruit in.

FRUIT JUICE SAUCE

½ pt. fruit juice
1 level dsp. arrowroot or cornflour

Blend the arrowroot with a little fruit juice. Add the rest of the juice and bring to the boil while stirring.

JELLIES

2 pts. of fruit juice or sieved fruit and juice
1¾ oz. gelatine

FRUIT FOOLS

Stew fruit in a little water and sugar. Liquidize or sieve fruit. Add fruit puree to a pint of thick custard. Add a little at a time, beat up thoroughly. To prevent a skin forming, cover top of fool with wet greaseproof and chill. Serve with shortbread.

PINEAPPLE UPSIDEDOWN PUDDING

1 tin of pineapple
1 oz. margarine
2 oz. sugar
2 tbs. golden syrup
7 oz. S.R. flour
1-1½ gill water
½ tsp. bicarb. soda

Drain pineapple rings into a sieve. Grease a pyrex dish thoroughly. Arrange pineapple in the bottom of the dish. Make eggless sponge: Cream margarine sugar, syrup together and beat until the mixture is very pale in colour. Dissolve soda in water. Add water and flour alternately to the creamed mixture stirring lightly. The mixture should be the consistency of thick batter. Pour mixture on to pineapple and bake for about 40 mins. in a moderately hot oven 350-375°F or Reg 4-5. Serve with custard or fruit juice sauce.

SHORTBREAD

3 oz. plain flour
1 oz. cornflour
3 oz. margarine
2 oz. sugar

Cream margarine and half the sugar. Work in the flour and the last of the sugar. Knead well. Press into a good round shape, place on back of tin or tray. Bake for 40 mins. in a slow oven 300-325°F/Reg 2. Cool on tin.

SUNFLOWER SHORTCAKE

4 oz. margarine
3 oz. Castor sugar
6 oz. Plain flour
1 medium size tin of peaches
2 round tsp. arrowroot

Cream together margarine and sugar until light and fluffy; beat in sieved flour until smooth. Grease an 8" sandwich tin. Press mixture into the tin and smooth top. Bake in moderate oven, 350°F/Reg 4. 25-30 mins. Remove and cool on wire tray. Drain peaches and slice thinly keeping half uncut for the centre. Measure ¼ pint juice. Arrange peach slices round edge of pastry, overlapping. Place uncut peach in centre. Blend arrowroot with fruit juice in a saucepan and bring to the boil. Boil for 2-3 mins. stirring continuously. Cool sauce slightly, coat fruit with arrowroot sauce. Leave to cool.

FLAPJACKS

6 oz. margarine
6 oz. demerara sugar
8 oz. porridge oats
Pinch of salt

Melt fat in saucepan over a gentle heat. Mix in sugar, oats and salt. Stir well, turn mixture into well greased tin and press lightly together. Smooth surface with a knife and bake for approx. 30-35 mins. in centre of a moderate oven 375°F or Reg. 4. When cooked to a golden brown, leave to cool for a few mins. Cut into squares or fingers. Leave in tin until quite cold before removing.

MELTING MOMENTS

3 oz. cornflour
1 oz. flour
3 oz. margarine
3-4 oz. icing sugar
Water

Cream together margarine and sugar. Sieve flour and cornflour together. Work into margarine mixture, then add a few drops of water to make a mixture that you can pipe or shape with fingers. Put into forcing bag and use a large piping rose. Alternatively shape into circles or oblongs with floured fingers on a greased baking tray. Bake for 15 mins. in the centre of a moderate oven 375°F/Reg. 4. Cool on tin. Sandwich together with butter icing.

VIENNESE TARTS

4 oz. margarine
1¼ oz. sieved icing sugar
2 oz. flour
2 oz. cornflour

Cream together margarine and icing sugar. Work in flour and cornflour, then pipe or spoon into small paper cases. Bake for about 45 mins. in very moderate oven for 40 mins. 350°F/Reg. 3 until pale brown. Fill centre with jam.

EGGLESS SANDWICH CAKE

1 oz. margarine
2 oz. sugar
2 tbs. golden syrup
Margarine icing
2 oz. icing sugar
7 oz. S.R. flour

1-1½ gils water
½ tsp. bicarb soda
1 tsp. coffee dissolved in a little water.

Cream fat, sugar and syrup. Dissolve soda in water. Add water and flour alternately to creamed mixture stirring lightly. The mixture should be the consistency of thick batter. Place mixture in a greased 8″ sandwich tin and bake for about 40 mins. in a moderately hot oven 350-375°F/Reg. 4-5. When cool, turn out and spread with coffee butter icing. Dissolve a heaped tsp. of instant coffee in a drop of water. Add to the creamed butter icing.

BANANA AND APRICOT (OR APPLE) LOAF

4 oz. margarine
5 oz. castor sugar
3 soft bananas
6 oz. S.R. flour
¼ tsp. bicarb. soda
3 oz. chopped dried apricot or apple
3 tbs. water

Grease 9″ loaf tin. Cream margarine and sugar until white and fluffy. Mash banana to a pulp. Add fruit and stir well. Add flour and bicarb. soda and water if the mixture is getting too stiff. The mixture should be a soft dropping consistency. Bake for 1 hour at 350°F or Reg. 4. Leave cake to cool in the tin.

APPENDIX III

Miscellaneous

NAMES OF SOME COMMONLY USED DRUGS

Antihistamines
Actidil
Anthisan
Benadryl
Co-Pyronil
Daneral-SA
Dibistin
Dilosyn
Dimotane LA
Fabahistin
Fenostil Retard
Histryl
Periactin
Phenergan
Piriton
Pro-Actidil
Tavegil
Thephorin
Triominic
Vallergan

Anti-Spasmodics
Aleudrin
Alupent
Amesec
Aminomed
Asmal
Asmapax

Bricanyl
Brontina
Brontisol
Brontrium
Brontyl
C.A.M.
Cardophylin
Choledyl
Englate
Entair
Etophylate
Expansyl
Felsol
Franol
Iso-Bronchisan
Isonien
Millophyline
Montheamin
Nethaprin Dospan
Neutraphylline
Numotac
Orthoxine
Silbe
Silbephylline
Spaneph
Taumasthman
Tedral
Thean

Theodrox
Theograd
Theo-Nar
Trentadil
Ventolin
Vortel

Aerosols
Becotide
Bextasol
Intal

Inhalers
Alupent
Bricanyl
Bronchilator
Brovon
Duo-Autohaler
Medihaler-Epi
Monotheamin & Amytal
PIB
Prenomiser
Pressurised Brovon
Pulmadil
Rybarex
Silbe
Ventolin

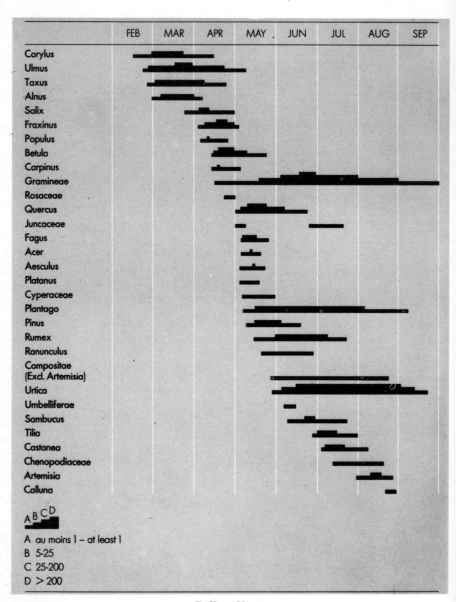

Pollen Chart

APPENDIX IV

Some sources of supplies and aids

DUST MASKS

These masks may be helpful when cleaning dusty areas, painting, or even cutting grass.

Surgical Face Masks (Johnson and Johnson)
Disposable Face Masks (Robinsons)

EXERCISES (BREATHING)

A booklet, *Exercises for Asthma and Emphysema,* is available from the Asthma Research Council, 12 Pembridge Square, London W.2.

NAME TAGS

Name tags should be worn by those who have drug, stinging-insect, or severe food allergies. They might prefer to carry a card in their wallet stating the substance to which they are allergic. Be certain to buy only stainless steel tags because others may turn green.

Necklaces are frequently lost, so bracelets are better. Girls may prefer a gold heart which can be engraved stating their name and type of allergy.

These may be obtained from Medic-Alert Foundation, 9 Hanover Street, London W.1.

Index